Fundamentals of Mammography

For Churchill Livingstone:

Editorial Director, Health Professions: Mary Law
Project Development Manager: Claire Wilson
Project Manager: Derek Robertson
Design Direction: Judith Wright

Fundamentals of Mammography

Linda Lee DCR MEd
Programme Leader, Postgraduate Certificate in Mammographic Studies,
Nottingham International Breast Education Centre, City Hospital, Nottingham, UK

Verdi Stickland TDCR
Radiographic Services Manager,
Nottingham International Breast Education Centre, City Hospital, Nottingham, UK

A Robin M Wilson MB ChB FRCR FRCP(E)
Associate Clinical Director and Consultant Radiologist,
Nottingham International Breast Education Centre, City Hospital, Nottingham, UK

Andrew Evans MB ChB MRCP FRCR
Consultant Radiologist,
Nottingham International Breast Education Centre, City Hospital, Nottingham, UK

Foreword by

Kristine M King MD
Radiologist and Medical Director, St Paul Radiology, St Paul, MN, USA

SECOND EDITION

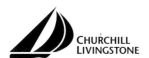

CHURCHILL
LIVINGSTONE

CHURCHILL LIVINGSTONE
An imprint of Elsevier Science Limited

First edition 1995
Second edition 2003

ISBN 0 443 071144

British Library Cataloguing in Publication Data
A catalogue record for this book is available from the British Library

Library of Congress Cataloging in Publication Data
A catalog record for this book is available from the Library of Congress

Note
Medical knowledge is constantly changing. As new information becomes
available, changes in treatment, procedures, equipment and the use of
drugs become necessary. The editors, contributors and the publishers have
taken care to ensure that the information given in this text is accurate and
up to date. However, readers are strongly advised to confirm that the
information, especially with regard to drug usage, complies with the latest
legislation and standards of practice.

The
publisher's
policy is to use
**paper manufactured
from sustainable forests**

Printed in China by RDC Group Limited

Contents

Foreword

Women coming in for mammograms place their trust in the technologists to obtain the best images possible so that potential cancer is detected early, when small and possibly curable. They are often anxious that an abnormality may be found. Patients with a new palpable lump are usually especially distressed on their arrival for evaluation. It is a never-ending challenge to comfort, calm, and educate these women as the work-up begins – whether it is special mammographic views, an ultrasound exam, or a biopsy.

Fundamental of Mammography remains the book of choice for mammography technologists who care about doing their best for the women they serve. This excellent book addresses both the technical and the human facets of this profession. There are explanations and clear diagrams that help technologists achieve the best images through positioning and an understanding of their equipment. These graphic aids show how to accommodate different statures, chest wall configurations, breast sizes, and varying breast tissue density, as well as how to achieve and maintain quality control for equipment and film processing. A section about procedures describes the different techniques for localization and biopsy, including types of equipment, the role of the technologist and potential complications associated with these procedures.

One chapter describes the benign and malignant features of various lesions and conditions in the breast, allowing technologists a better understanding of these disease processes. This will also better equip them to understand what is needed in the way of imaging and to understand why radiologists may ask them to obtain certain special views. There is an entire chapter dedicated to these 'complementary projections'. A discussion of male mammography is also included in this section.

This book goes beyond mere technical instruction. The anxieties of these women, with or without a problem, are very real. All who work in this field know that mammography is one of the most emotionally charged areas of medicine. Chapter 13, *Psychological Issues and Communication*, is dedicated to helping dissipate this emotional tension through education, communication, and understanding.

This classic has also been updated in its layout: for quick reference, there is a section on the first page of each chapter that lays out the contents of the chapter. The text has also been updated to reflect changes in technology since the first edition. This thorough, instructional book, which does an excellent job of addressing both the technical and psychological aspects of this field, remains the preferred text for technologists in mammography as well as for those who are involved in the instruction of technologists.

Kristine M King, MD

Preface

High quality mammography is essential in the fight against breast cancer, whether it be as a method of screening or as part of the assessment of women with breast symptoms.

The quality of a mammogram depends on:

- the clinical environment,
- the communication skills of the radiographer,
- the technical skills of the radiographer,
- the quality and performance of the equipment and, above all,
- the dedication of the radiographer.

The aim of this book is to assist the radiographer performing mammography to deliver a consistently high quality service. We believe that a knowledgeable radiographer is in the best posi-

tion to do so. To this end this book goes beyond what is traditionally regarded as appropriate for a radiographer to know. Radiographers must have an understanding not only of the technical and physical aspects of mammograpy but also of why mammography is performed and how it is interpreted. A good mammographer will be able to use this knowledge to apply initiative and provide the radiologist with the information required for accurate and clinically relevant mammographic diagnosis.

Linda Lee
Verdi Stickland
A. Robin M. Wilson
Eric J. Roebuck

Abbreviations

AEC   automatic exposure control/chamber
ANDI   aberrations of normal development and involution
BBC   benign breast changes
CAD   computer-aided diagnosis
COSHH   Control of Substances Hazardous to Health
DCIS   ductel carcinoma in situ
FNA   fine needle aspiration
HIP   Health Insurance Plan
HRT   hormone replacement therapy
LBD   light beam diaphragm
LCIS   lobular carcinoma in situ
NHS   National Health Service
NHSBSP National Health Service Breast Screening Programme
OD   optical density
PPV   positive predictive value
QA   quality assurance
TDL   terminal ductolobular unit
TQM   total quality management
U/S   ultrasound

1

Mammography equipment and quality control

This chapter outlines:
- the basic requirements of mammography equipment,
- routine quality control testing.

INTRODUCTION

The purchase, commissioning and quality control of equipment is essential to the provision of a quality mammographic service. Without careful consideration of the factors outlined in this and the next chapter, the technical expertise of the mammographer will be wasted and the diagnostic information available to the skilled radiologist reduced.

MAMMOGRAPHIC EQUIPMENT CHOICE

Design

The equipment chosen for mammography must be acceptable to both the operator and the woman to be examined. It must be easy to use and, especially in the screening situation, should be light to manipulate. Large, unwieldy equipment is usually physically demanding on the operators who have to use it and may be frightening to the woman being examined. It should not appear threatening to the women and to this end its ergonomic design is all important. Even the colour choice made by the manufacturer should be carefully thought out; pastel colours, for example, appear to be less threatening than harsh primary colours. All areas of the equipment which come into contact with the woman must be smooth, with no sharp edges or corners, and no external parts should become excessively hot.

Most women are able to stand while mammography is performed but handles must be available at appropriate levels to allow the unsteady or frail to hold on without compromising the accurate positioning of the breast and adjacent pectoralis major muscle.

The perfect mammography unit has not yet been designed from the point of view of either the operator or the patient. Some designs are better than others, but choosing equipment always involves compromise.

Functional requirements

It is important that the machine is able to perform to a consistently high standard over time. Very small changes in the breast may be the only indication that there is a developing cancer. Mammography provides a mechanism for early detection but the equipment must be reliable and consistent in its performance. It should be robust enough to cope with in excess of 300 exposures per day.

The following equipment parameters must be considered:

- high-voltage generator,
- kV output,
- tube current,
- focal spot size,
- automatic exposure control device,
- grid.

High-voltage generator

This must supply a near DC high voltage. Any ripple should be less than 5%.

From 2003 the voltage limits imposed on the electricity supply companies in the UK will be increased to ±10%. It is essential that equipment will function correctly from the supply voltage. Since supply losses increase with the distance from the transformer this is particularly relevant to equipment installed on trailers which will operate from various mains outlets.

kV output

Most modern mammography machines have a generator providing constant potential. The high voltage applied to the tube must be from 22 to 35 kV in increments of 1 kV, accurate to ± 1 kV. A voltage of 22 kV accommodates imaging biopsy specimens. Most up-to-date mammography units have a facility for automatic selection of the kV to optimize contrast or dose this is achieved in most cases by the target and filtration materials automatically selected to provide the optimum wave-form.

Tube current (mA)

Tube current should be as high as possible to keep exposure times to a minimum thus reducing the risk of movement blur. The current at 28 kV should be at least 100 mA on large focus, with limits of ±10%, and 30 mA with similar limits on small focus.

Focal spot size

The focal spot should be as small as possible, nominally 0.3 mm (large focus) for routine mammography and no more that a nominal 0.1 mm (small focus) for magnification views.

Automatic exposure control (AEC) device

An accurate automatic exposure control device is essential. The AEC detector must be movable, from both sides of the support table, so that it may underlie the most dense area of the breast, usually some 2 cm behind the nipple. The position of the device must be clearly indicated to the operator. To allow for anatomical variations, the device should move from 2 cm to 12 cm from the chest wall edge of the breast support table. The AEC device must be capable of being preset to at least two levels, to allow for differing film/screen combinations. The machine should also allow the operator to adjust the resulting density levels, to compensate for any changes in film sensitivity and for changes in processing parameters. This should be in steps of 5–10%. It should compensate for changes in thickness of breast tissue in the range of 2 to 10 cm with an accuracy of ±0.15 OD.

Grid

A moving grid, with 4:1 or 5:1 ratio, is essential to good image quality despite the increased dose this requires. The grid factor should be less than 2.5 at 30 kV. The mechanism to move the grid should be designed so that no grid lines are seen under any exposure conditions.

POST-INSTALLATION PROCEDURES

A critical inspection, carried out by competent, qualified engineers, is mandatory in order to ensure that the equipment has been delivered and installed according to specification and to confirm complete electrical safety. Independent quality control medical physicists should then carry out commissioning and acceptance tests. These tests should follow clearly defined and recognized guidelines such as those defined by the United Kingdom Institute of Physical Sciences in Medicine.

Before any mammography is undertaken a radiographer should check that the equipment is functioning satisfactorily and that it is safe. A radiographer, at commissioning, and at regular intervals should carry out the following safety checks thereafter.

- There should be no sharp edges.
- The emergency power switch should work quickly and easily.
- The compression should be released on emergency switch-off.
- There should be no powered movement of the breast support table when compression is applied.
- There should be the capability to override the automatic release of compression after exposure (for use during localizations using a perforated plate or co-ordinate grid plate).
- The maximum compression force should be limited to 200 newtons (20 kg).
- The light within the light beam diaphragm (LBD) should remain on for no longer than 120 seconds and the area surrounding the LBD should not feel unduly hot to the woman, should she come into contact with it.
- All mechanical movements should be free running and all brakes should function correctly. There should be no overrun of any movement following release of the drive switch.
- All accessories should attach easily and securely. There should be no risk of injury to the operator or to the woman being examined.

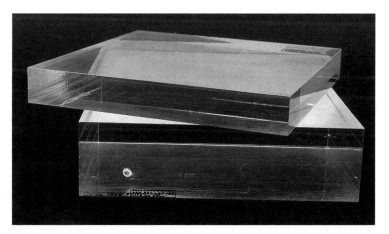

Figure 1.1   Perspex blocks for quality control tests.

ROUTINE DAILY EQUIPMENT PERFORMANCE MONITORING

Before testing, the equipment should be warmed up according to the manufacturer's instructions. The output (mAs) should be checked daily and remain consistent from day to day.

Equipment required for quality control testing of the mammography system

- Perspex block 4 cm thick (this mimics the absorption of the 'standard' breast),
- perspex block 2 cm thick (**Figure 1.1**),
- designated cassette – clearly identified,
- mammography film from the current batch,
- image quality phantom (**Figure 1.2**).

Testing the AEC device

These tests are carried out following the normal daily warm-up procedure as recommended by the manufacturer.

Consistency The 4 cm block of perspex is placed on the breast support table, slightly overlapping the chest wall edge and covering the AEC chamber, which should be in the chest wall position. The empty test cassette is then placed in the bucky, the machine set to the normal setting used for mammography and an exposure made. The post-exposure mAs reading is noted. This procedure is repeated three times, noting the post-exposure mAs reading each time. These readings should not vary more than 5% of the expected value and no machine should vary by more than 10%.

Reproducibility The cassette is loaded with the film in current use for mammography and a further exposure made. This post-exposure mAs reading is logged and the film processed. Using a densitometer, the optical density on the film is measured at a point 4 cm from the chest wall edge in the mid-line. This reading should also be logged. The optical density (OD) achieved should not vary more than 0.15 OD from the norm for the system. The normal base density for the 4 cm block should fall within the range 1.4–1.8 OD.

The results from these tests should be displayed in graphic form to ensure that trends are quickly identified and steps taken to rectify an adverse situation before there is deterioration in the quality of the mammograms (**Figure 1.3**). This test should be repeated daily. The limiting values should be agreed with the radiologist in charge of the unit after consultation with the medical physics department. No mammography should be undertaken when the test results exceed these values.

Thickness compensation To check for consistency of the AEC with varying densities of breast tissue, the above tests should be repeated weekly using perspex blocks of 2, 4 and 6 or 7 cm thicknesses. The post-exposure mAs readings should not vary more than 10% from week to week for each thickness of perspex. The resulting optical densities should not vary more than 0.15 OD for

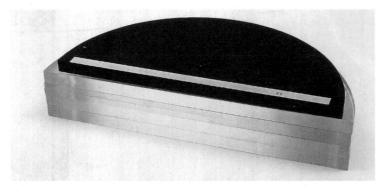

Figure 1.2 An image quality phantom.

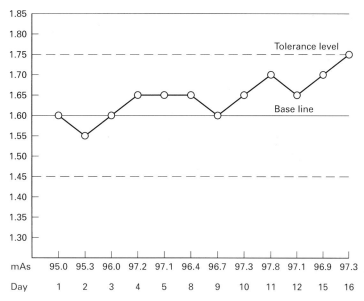

Figure 1.3 4 cm block densities. See text for explanation.

each thickness. A change in mAs value may indicate that the x-ray tube voltage has altered.

Testing image quality

Image quality should be checked using an image quality test phantom (see **Figure 1.2**). This test will assess the whole system, including the imaging system. The test object should be used according to the manufacturer's instruction manual. A film should be taken weekly of the image test phantom and compared with the 'gold standard' film which was made on installation of the equipment. The test should be repeated following any servicing or repair of the equipment or when a problem is suspected.

Testing cassettes

When the system is set up, all the new cassettes should be tested for speed, film/screen contact and light tightness. The screens should be cleaned with a proprietary anti-static screen cleaner and allowed to dry before the cassettes are loaded. The cassettes should be loaded with the mammography film in current use and it is recommended that they are allowed to rest for

10 minutes before exposing in the bucky using the 4 cm block of perspex. Allowing the cassettes to rest ensures that any air trapped in the cassette dissipates and does not give a false result. The post-exposure mAs readout should be noted and the resulting optical densities should be measured as described previously. The mAs readings for each cassette should be within 5% of the mean value. The resulting optical densities should be within 0.10 OD of the mean value.

The cassettes should now be reloaded and placed on top of the breast support table with a mammography film screen test grid placed directly on top (Gammex RMI 318B is suitable). An exposure is made, sufficient to result in an optical density of 2.0 OD measured in the density spot on the chest wall edge. The film is processed and viewed at a distance of approximately 1 metre. If there is poor film/screen contact in any area it will show as an area of increased density. If there are any such areas, the screens are recleaned, the cassettes reloaded and the test repeated after an interval to confirm the presence of a fault.

The test for light leakage is the standard one described in Appendix A of BS7534:1991, IEC 406 1975. The cassette is loaded with mammography film and then exposed to the light from a 100 watt tungsten filament lamp at a distance of 1 metre for 10 minutes. This is repeated for each of the six surfaces of the cassette. The film is processed and examined for areas of fogging. Any cassettes showing any fault should be rejected and returned to the manufacturer for replacement. It is important when cassettes are replaced that they match the existing ones. The screens should be numbered and the cassettes identified with the same number before being put into service.

The cassette tests should be repeated quarterly and the results noted in a log book. Cassettes and screens should be cleaned each day before being used, using a proprietary anti-static cleaner.

STEREOTACTIC DEVICES

Stereotactic devices, if seldom used, should be tested before each use or weekly if in constant use. This is carried out using a suitable test object which usually consists of a perspex block with drilled holes of differing depths. These are generally supplied by the equipment manufacturer. When the test object used is a perspex block then the test should be repeated for more than one drilled hole, or for more than one object when a wax phantom is used.

Testing stereotactic devices

The stereotactic device is installed according to the manufacturer's instructions. The phantom is placed on the breast support table in the position that the breast would occupy, ensuring that the AEC chamber is in the chest wall position. The procedure will then vary depending whether the unit is digital or not. For film/screen two exposures are made with the tube swung through 15 degrees to either side, according to the manufacturer's instructions. The film is processed and placed on the digitizer. For small field digital an initial scout exposure will be required.

Following the instructions pertinent to the equipment, the device is localized over one of the holes in the phantom. The needle guide is placed in the position required to insert a needle in the chosen hole, a needle is installed and a further two exposures are made, to check the position of the needle tip. The above procedure is then repeated, selecting another hole in the phantom. When the needle tip does not reach the bottom of the selected holes then the stereotactic device is out of calibration and an engineer should be called to recalibrate the device. One major manufacturer provides instructions and tools for the operator to recalibrate the stereotactic device without the need to call upon the services of an engineer. In this case, the instructions for recalibrating should be followed and the check sequence repeated.

FURTHER READING

American Association of Physicists in Medicine. *Equipment Requirements and Quality Control for Mammography*. AAPM Report 29. New York: American Institute of Physics, 1990.

American College of Radiology. *American Mammography Quality Control Manual* (August 2000).

Andolina VF, Lille SL, Willison KM. *Mammography Imaging: a Practical Guide*. Philadelphia: JB Lippincott, 2001 2nd edition.

Barnes GT, Frey DG. *Screen Film Mammography: Imaging Considerations and Medical Physics Responsibilities*. Madison: Medical Physics Publishing, 1991.

Department of Health. *Guidelines on the Establishment of a Quality Assurance System for the Radiological Aspects of Mammography used for Breast Screening*. Report of a sub-committee of the Radiological Advisory Committee of the Chief Medical Officer. London: Department of Health, 1989.

European Guidelines for Quality Assurance in Mammography Screening (2000) Luxembourg: Office for Official Publications of the European Communities.

Farria DM, Bassett LW, Kimme-Smith C, DeBruhl N. Mammographic quality assurance from A to Z. *Radiographics* 1994; **14**: 371–385.

Institute of Physical Sciences in Medicine (IPSM). *The Commissioning and Routine Testing of Mammography X-ray Systems*. Report no. 59. York: IPSM, 1994.

Kimme-Smith C. New and future developments in screen–film mammography equipment and techniques. *Radiological Clinics of North America* 1992; **30**: 55–66.

Kimme-Smith C, Bassett LW, Gold RH. *Workbook for Quality Mammography*, 2nd edition. Williams & Wilkins, 1997.

Lawinski C, Young K, Hancock C. *Guidance Notes for the Evaluation of Mammographic X-ray Equipment*. Sheffield: NHSBSP Publications, 1997.

Long SM. *Handbook of Mammography*, 4th edition. Mammography Consulting Services Ltd, 2000.

Medical Devices Agency. Evaluation Report MDA 01011. *Further Revisions To Guidance Notes For Health Authorities and NHS Trusts on Mammographic X-ray Equipment For Breast Screening*. HMSO, 2001.

National Health Service Breast Screening Programme. *A Radiographic Quality Control Manual for Mammography*. Sheffield: NHSBSP Publications, 1999.

Nielsen B. Technical aspects of mammography. *Current Opinion in Radiology* 1992; **4**: 118–122.

Wentz G. *Mammography for Radiologic Technologists*. New York: McGraw Hill, 1992.

2

Film processing and quality control

This chapter outlines how to:
- carry out film processing tests,
- monitor the consistency of the imaging system.

INTRODUCTION

Digital imaging will be the method of recording breast mammography in the future. Films with intensifying screens are currently the imaging system of choice. Xerography can no longer be recommended due to the inherent increase in radiation dose and poor contrast gradient.

The film almost exclusively used at present for mammography has a single emulsion coated on one side of the base with an anti-halation backing on the reverse. This emulsion is at its most sensitive in the green region of the visible spectrum. This spectral sensitivity is closely matched to the light emission from the single fluorescent screen in the mammography cassette.

Film choice is dependent to a degree on the preference of the radiologist responsible for reading the films, but certain criteria must be considered when making this choice. The breast consists of soft tissue which has low inherent radiographic contrast. The characteristics of the film used must therefore include a combination of high contrast and, to keep radiation dose to a minimum, high speed.

Mammography film is particularly sensitive to variations in processing parameters. It is important that the films are processed in a machine where the parameters are closely controlled and monitored. Extended processing has been recommended with a development time of 35–40 seconds at a temperature of 32–35 degrees C but developments in film technology have allowed the more common use of rapid processing. Dedicated processing is recommended but only in units where there is sufficient throughput of films to maintain processor stability; fewer than 25 films per day for the average processor is unlikely to be sufficient. The heated developer will oxidize and one tank volume of replenisher must be added to the tank to overcome this effect. In addition, to reach equilibrium with new chemical reagents, the system will require a further three tank volumes of replenisher or the addition of a suitable starter specific to mammography. The larger the developer tank capacity, the greater the throughput necessary to keep the system stable. Even with a small capacity system this is very difficult to achieve.

Once optimum processing conditions have been achieved it is vitally important that they are maintained for the production of consistent quality images. To this end the processing must be carefully monitored and controlled. A quality control programme should be established and rigidly adhered to.

All radiographers should be aware of the regulations relating to COSHH (Control of Substances Hazardous to Health). More manufacturers are using gluteraldehyde-free developer to improve health and safety. Care must be taken to ensure that the rollers in the processor are kept clean and in good condition as with this type of developer the emulsion is more vulnerable to physical damage.

Equipment required for testing film processing

- A 21 step light sensitometer,
- densitometer of proven accuracy or a QC system such as Pehmed or Windense (**Figure 2.1**)
- thermometer (not mercury as there is a risk of contamination should it break),
- processor control charts (**Figure 2.2**),
- measuring jug,

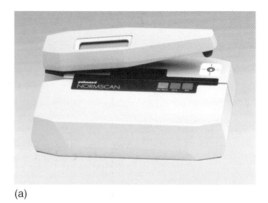

(a)

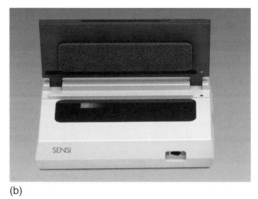

(b)

Figure 2.1 Pehamed system.

- a dedicated box of mammography film with the same batch number as those in current use for mammograms.

Method of testing

To initiate a quality control programme standard baselines must first be established:

- The processor must be allowed to attain its normal working temperature.
- Under suitable safe-light conditions, and using the green setting on the sensitometer, a sheet of film from the dedicated box of film is exposed by placing it emulsion side down in the sensitometer. The film is processed in such a way that the least dense step of the image enters the tank first. This is important as it avoids changes in the density of the steps due to changes in the temperature and activity of the chemical reagents in the tank.

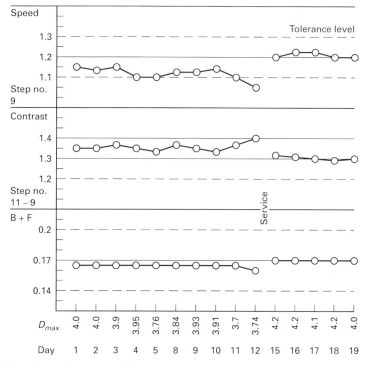

Figure 2.2   An example of a processor control chart.

(With most daylight loading systems the film enters the processor with a long edge leading. It is therefore important that the density strip is placed on the same edge of the film each time.)

- The temperature of the developer is noted. If the processor has a readout of proven accuracy this can be used, but failing this, the thermometer should be used to read the temperature of the developer immediately after processing the film. To do this the thermometer should be placed in the developer tank at the same point each time at a place remote from the replenisher inlet.
- The densitometer is zeroed.

Using a manual densitometer the following readings should be taken from the film strip and written on the film using a marker pen.

Base + fog   This is the lowest density achievable on the chosen film when processed through that processor using the chosen chemical reagents and processing conditions.

An unexposed area on the film is measured. This gives the value of base + fog (B+F). This value is noted on the film with a marker pen. It should be less than 0.20 OD.

Speed index   The centre of the step which gives a value of 1.0 OD above B+F is measured. This should be in the centre of the straight line portion of the characteristic curve for the film under the chosen processing conditions. This value and step number are noted on the film. This gives the speed index of the film.

Contrast   Film contrast is important as it allows small density differences in the breast to be visualized. It is a measure of the steepness of the slope of the straight line portion of the characteristic curve.

The centre of the step which has an optical density of approximately 2.0 OD is measured. This value and step number is noted on the film. The value of the speed step is subtracted from this value. This determines the contrast of the film. The contrast value is noted on the film.

Maximum density (*D*max) *D*max is important for viewing films as it is the density of the background of the film.

The step with the highest density value is measured (this may not be step 21). The value and step number are noted on the film.

The same identified steps must always be used.

Reference values

To establish reference values the whole operation is repeated a further nine times and the mean calculated by averaging the values. This should be done within the space of 2 days. The step numbers and the reference values are noted on a processor control chart. Now that the reference values have been established, the processor can be monitored.

On the processor control chart (**Figure 2.2**) the **step numbers** which are to be used to monitor processing are noted. The **tolerance values** allowed are marked on the chart above and below the reference values.

Limits of acceptability

The following are the generally accepted limits of acceptability:

- The value of **base + fog** should be less than 0.20 OD. Depending on the choice of film a value of 0.17 OD is easily achievable. Limits of acceptability on this are ± 0.03 OD.
- For the **speed index** the limit should be ± 0.10 OD.
- For **contrast** the limit should be ± 0.10 OD.
- For **Dmax** the minimum acceptable level is 3.6 OD. This high level is required to maintain the observer's ability to see small variations in density within the image by excluding all light from the background of the mammogram.

PROCESSOR MONITORING

Each day, when the processor has attained its normal working levels, a sensitometry strip should be exposed and processed in the manner just described and the readings recorded on the chart. When the readings fall outwith the agreed tolerances the first step to take is to make another sensitometry strip. When this also produces readings which are out of tolerance, then corrective action must be taken. Until the processor returns to stable levels no mammograms should be processed through it. Daily chart recording will usually show adverse trends and will allow corrective action to be taken well before the system exceeds tolerance levels.

The computer-based systems when used to monitor the strips automatically record the data and calculate the speed and gamma of the film.

The following additional information should be recorded on the processor monitoring chart:

- Chemical reagent changes. When the chemicals in the tanks have been changed this information should be recorded on the chart and the points on the graph following this should not be joined to those previously recorded.
- New box of films. To ensure that it is the processor which is being monitored and not the whole imaging system, it is necessary to perform a crossover by using a film from the old box and one from the new and processing them together. These films should be compared to ensure that the readings on both coincide. If they do not match, the film batch numbers should be checked; if the batch numbers match, the test should be repeated. Film box changes and batch numbers should be marked on the processor control chart.

Processor servicing and cleaning

The date when this takes place should be recorded. The processor should be monitored before and after servicing. This post-service check should be done before the engineer leaves the department.

Other checks which should be done are as follows.

Replenishment

The machine should maintain constant activity of the chemicals by continuously topping up the tank with fresh chemical reagents. The checking of this should be undertaken following the manufacturer's instructions. The replenishment rate required will depend on the use of the processor. The area of film processed and the work load will all affect this as will the average densities of the films being processed.

Replenishment rates will be checked by the service engineer at routine service but may have to be repeated in the interval if a persistent problem is identified. If activity of the chemical reagents drops, as indicated by a reduction in the **speed index**, this may be due to failure in the replenishment pump.

Replenishment rates should remain within 5% of the values set at the last service visit. It is important that the chemicals are mixed according to the manufacturer's instructions because there may be precipitation in the replenisher tanks if there is not enough water in the tank when certain of the chemicals are added. It is useful to monitor the amount of chemical reagents being used by the processor as this can give an indication of a problem when demand falls off while the work load remains constant.

Fixer replenishment is also important. The time taken to fix the film will double by the time the level of silver in the tank reaches 3 g/l. Silver levels can be measured by using silver estimating papers. Fixer replenishment rates should be increased when the level of silver in the tank becomes too high. However, too high a rate of replenishment will mean that there will be inefficient use of chemical reagents.

Processor cycle time

Any variation in the time which the film spends in the developer tank results in a change of blackening on the film. This affects **base + fog**, the **speed index** and **contrast**. Cycle time should be measured on installation of the processor to obtain a baseline value and should be repeated before and after routine servicing. It should be repeated when there is a problem with film density. The time it takes from the leading edge of the film entering the processor to the same edge emerging from the drier is measured, using a stopwatch or a watch with a second sweep. The time taken for the film to pass through the processor should not vary by more than 5 seconds from the time set.

Developer temperature

Developer temperature is a critical factor in film processing. A variation of less than 1 degrees C may result in a significant density variation on the film. On installation the accuracy of the temperature indicator should be established and this should be regularly checked. A digital or alcohol-filled thermometer should be used to measure the developer tank temperature at the same point in the tank (away from the replenisher inlet) and the result compared with the displayed value. This should be repeated until accuracy of the readout has been established. (A mercury-filled thermometer should not be used. There is a risk of contamination should a breakage occur). Developer tank temperature should vary by less than 0.5 degrees C in normal use.

Any change in the pH or **specific gravity** of the chemical reagents may result in processing changes. These may be checked using pH papers and a hydrometer. Values for these are specific to the chemical manufacturer but should be pH 10–11 for developer and pH 4–5 for fixer. The manufacturer will specify the limiting factors.

Silver recovery

In these ecologically conscious days silver recovery is important. Silver estimating papers can be used to measure the level of silver in the spent fixer. In the UK it is necessary to seek the permission of the local water authority before dumping spent chemical reagents in the sewer. The level of silver allowed in the effluent will depend on the local licensing authority and is dependent on the amount of water flowing at the same time as the spent chemical reagents.

Residual spent reagents

To check the efficiency of the washing process a chemical test will indicate whether all the chemical reagents have been removed from the processed film. Staining of the stored mammogram will result if the washing process is inadequate. The temperature of the wash water should be between 18 and 20 degrees C to achieve archival permanence. Maintenance of the processor should be undertaken according to the manufacturer's instructions. Rollers require special attention as dirty or worn rollers will cause marks on the films. Care should be taken when cleaning the rollers that the pad used to scrub them is not too harsh.

FURTHER READING

Andolina VF, Lille SL, Willison KM. *Mammography Imaging: a practical guide*. Philadelphia: JB Lippincott, 2001.

Barnes GT, Frey DG. *Screen Film Mammography: Imaging Considerations and Medical Physics Responsibilities*. Madison: Medical Physics Publishing, 1991.

Farria DM, Bassett LW, Kimme-Smith C, DeBruhl N. Mammographic quality assurance from A to Z. *Radiographics* 1994; **14**: 371–385.

Moores BM, Watkinson SA, Henshaw ET, Pearcy BJ. *Practical Guide to Quality Assurance in Medical Imaging*. Chichester: John Wiley & Sons, 1987.

National Health Service Breast Screening Programme. *A Radiographic Quality Control Manual for Mammography*. Sheffield, NHSBSP Publications, 1999.

Nielsen B. Technical aspects of mammography. *Current Opinion in Radiology* 1992; **4**: 118–122.

Tanner RL. Mammography unit compression force: acceptance test and quality control protocols. *Radiology* 1992; **184**: 45–48.

Wentz G. *Mammography for Radiologic Technologists*. New York: McGraw Hill, 1992.

3

Breast anatomy – implications for mammographic practice

This chapter provides an outline of:

- the embryology of the breast,
- normal breast development and activity,
- mammographic involution,
- interruptions to the involutionary process,
- the anatomy of the adult breast,
- commonly encountered congenital anomalies,
- the development of breast cancer,
- anatomically derived mammographic principles.

EMBRYOLOGY

Every human embryo, both male and female, develops a ridge of tissue on each side of the body

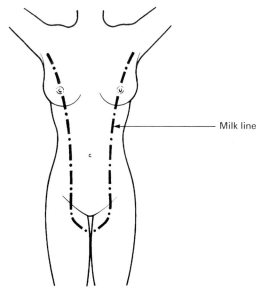

Figure 3.1   The milk line, running from clavicle to groin.

Milk line

which runs from the clavicular region to the groin along the 'milk line' (**Figure 3.1**). These are the lactogenic ridges, and it is from these ridges that the breast tissue develops. Most of the tissue forming the ridges atrophies and disappears during embryonic life, leaving a single island on each side of the chest. Each of these develops into a rudimentary breast which persists throughout infancy and childhood. Occasionally total atrophy of the remaining tissue does not occur and other islands of breast tissue persist at other sites along the lactogenic ridges. In this eventuality accessory breast tissue will develop in the adult. Development of the accessory tissue may be complete and a separate accessory breast will be formed. More usually, the development is incomplete and the only evience in the adult is an accessory nipple or simply a mole-like abnormality on the skin.

NORMAL DEVELOPMENT
Normal development

Glandular tissue

About 15–20 rods of tissue grow down from the apex of the island of lactogenic tissue into the rudimentary tissue beneath. The rods branch successively as they penetrate deeply, and ultimately become hollow. These are the breast ducts. The terminal portions of the branching system are where the functioning breast tissues form. The terminal ducts branch into ductules from which buds grow. These buds open out to form lobules, the epithelial-lined cavities which are the milk-producing glandular elements of the breast. A terminal duct and the associated lobules arising from it are called the terminal ductolobular unit (TDL). These TDLs are the most important part of the breast, from the point of view of both normal physiological function and the development of breast disease. Not only do most benign conditions have their origin in this area, but it is from the epithelial cells lining the TDLs that breast cancers arise.

Postnatal development

In females the hormonal influences of puberty cause further development of the rudimentary

breast tissues. Increased branching of the duct system leads to an increase in the number of TDLs. The TDLs themselves increase in size by proliferation in the number and size of the epithelial cells lining each lobular cavity and by expansion of the ductal and lobular lamina.

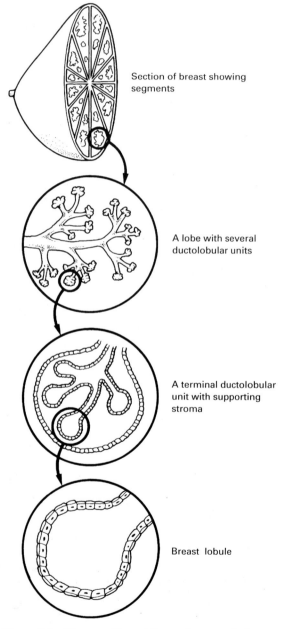

Section of breast showing segments

A lobe with several ductolobular units

A terminal ductolobular unit with supporting stroma

Breast lobule

Figure 3.2 Diagram of breast tissue at progressively increasing magnifications.

Approximately 20% of adolescent boys also experience some degree of breast development (gynaecomastia) which is usually transient.

On a mammogram each TDL casts a shadow about 1 mm in diameter. When development is complete, at around the age of 20 years, there are many hundreds of TDLs completely filling the breast. Superimposition of the TDL shadows forms the uniform overall density of the breast seen on mammography.

The breast is divided into 15–20 segments or lobes. Each segment contains a network of ducts that drain the TDLs. Under the nipple these ducts coalesce to form lactiferous sinuses which, in turn, drain out through the nipple. In the breast there are fibrous septa (ligaments of Astley Cooper) that divide and support the segments. The tissue within each segment is of two types: glandular tissue supported in a stroma of fibrofatty tissue (**Figure 3.2**).

Accessory breast tissue

It is not uncommon for the islands of glandular tissue developing in the lactogenic ridges to grow in two parts, with an additional small col-

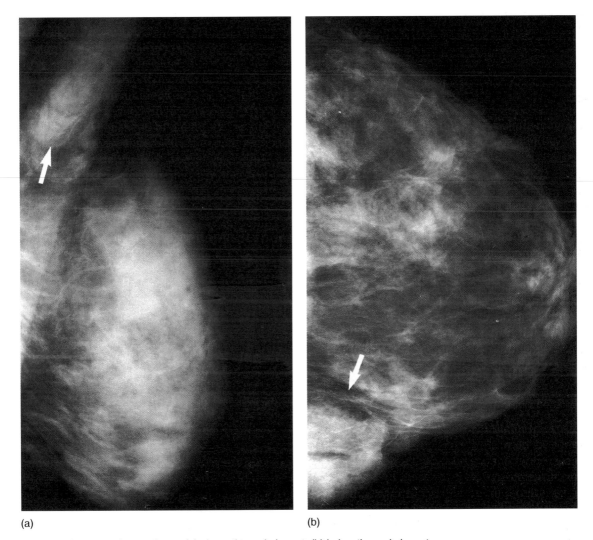

(a)   (b)

Figure 3.3   Accessory breast tissue: (a) above the main breast; (b) below the main breast.

lection immediately adjacent to the main island of tissue, usually above but sometimes below. Although the development of accessory breast tissue is usually bilateral, it is not always symmetrical, and may be unilateral. The accessory breast tissue can be visualized on a mammogram as a separate island of normal-looking glandular tissue lying within the breast (**Figure 3.3a,b**). The condition may be noticed as a palpable mass by a woman or her clinician, but the anxiety generated by this discovery is readily relieved on inspection of the mammogram.

NORMAL ACTIVITY

From maturity to the menopause, with interruptions for pregnancy, there are, associated with each menstrual cycle, alternating increases and decreases in the size and activity of the epithelial cells lining each TDL.

The cyclical increases and decreases are not usually associated with any perceptible change in mammographic appearance. It may, however, be difficult for a radiographer to obtain adequate compression if a breast is tender during the premenstrual phase. In this situation a mammogram may be of inferior quality and will therefore appear different, being more dense than one taken with proper compression. Should a radiographer encounter difficulties in examining a woman in the premenstrual part of her cycle, then the examination may be best deferred until mid-cycle. For the same reason, if a woman has suffered undue discomfort or pain during a mammographic examination in the past, future examinations are better scheduled to be undertaken in mid-cycle.

MAMMOGRAPHIC INVOLUTION

It is important not to confuse a mammographic appearance of a dense or fatty breast pattern with the process of physiological involution. The density of the breast tissues on mammography depends upon a number of factors: the amount of glandular tissue, the amount of fibrous tissue, and the degree of obesity of the woman. Some 20% of women at age 30 have a fatty appearance, and

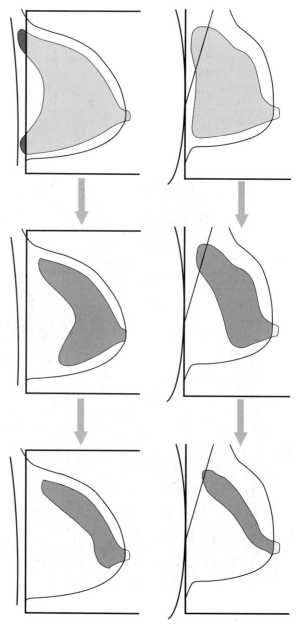

Figure 3.4   Process of mammographic involution.

approximately 40% of 80-year-olds have a dense pattern.

Physiological involution of the breast glandular tissue starts virtually as soon as a woman is mature, and can be regarded as the reverse of development. The TDLs decrease in size, eventually being replaced by fibrous tissue and fat. This process is quite different from the concept of mammographic involution.

Mammographic involution is the process of progressive reduction in the density of breast tissue. This is associated with a reduction in the proportion of the breast which is occupied by that density and also the change in shape of the dense portion. This process may be obscured completely in a breast with a high fibrous tissue content.

Evidence of mammographic involution is seen initially in the periphery of the breast, noted on a mammogram as an increase in the size of the layer of fat in the subcutaneous and retromammary regions. The breast tissue densities then start to shrink and finally disappear. The tissues in the lower inner quadrant change more rapidly than those in the upper inner and lower outer quadrants, with those in the superolateral quadrant usually the last to show change (**Figure 3.4**). By the age when routine mammography is indicated, mammographic involution of the breast is reasonably well advanced, particularly inferiorly and medially. The residual visible uninvoluted disc of glandular tissue density is then orientated in an oblique plane extending from behind the nipple upwards into the axillary tail, surrounded by a layer of fatty tissue (**Figure 3.5**). Lundgren recognized the importance of the orientation of the glandular breast

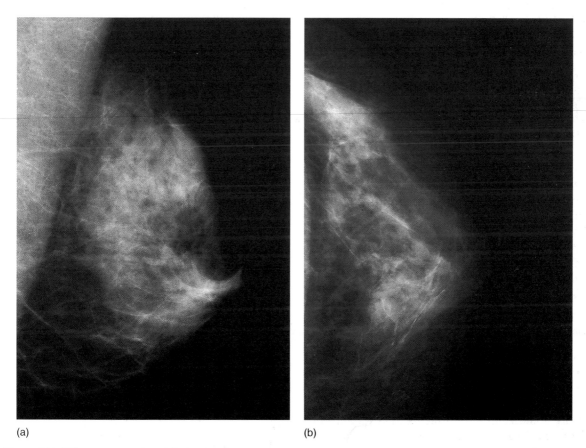

(a)   (b)

Figure 3.5   Mammograms of partially involuted breast showing oblique orientation of uninvoluted tissue: (a) medio-lateral oblique projection; (b) cranio-caudal projection.

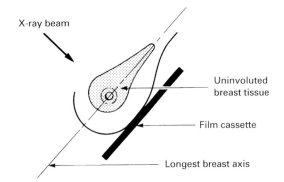

Figure 3.6 The medio-lateral oblique projection illustrating maximal demonstration of breast tissue without foreshortening.

tissue and was the first to recognize the value of the medio-lateral oblique projection (**Figure 3.6**). The advantages of this projection are now universally accepted.

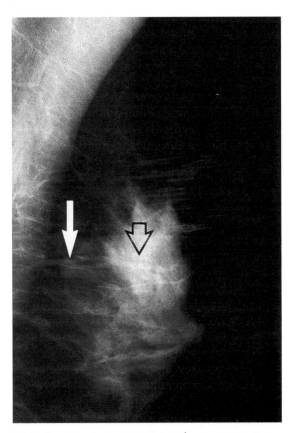

Figure 3.7 Mammogram indicating (↓) correct and incorrect (+) positioning of the automatic exposure device.

Mammographic involution also has a fundamental bearing on the choice of position of the automatic exposure chamber (AEC) of the mammography table. The AEC should be positioned under a dense portion of the breast rather than an area of fat. If this position cannot be assessed from a study of previous mammograms, then a point some 3–5 cm above and behind the nipple should be selected (**Figure 3.7**).

INTERRUPTIONS TO THE INVOLUTIONARY PROCESS
Pregnancy

With pregnancy each TDL hypertrophies to become larger than the size achieved during normal cyclical activity. Simultaneously the ducts dilate and the whole breast will appear very dense on a mammogram. Mammography should only be performed in exceptional circumstances during pregnancy. Following the cessation of lactation the breast reverts to the pre-pregnancy appearance within a few weeks. Thereafter the slow disappearance of glandular density continues at the same rate as before the pregnancy.

Hormone replacement therapy

In the last few years the numbers of women taking Hormone Replacement Therapy (HRT) has increased significantly. Two questions have been raised about the use of HRT.

Influence on breast density

The use of HRT can impact on the mammographic density of the breast. Effectively it represses, and to some degree reverses, the mammographic involutionary process. The impact of HRT on breast patterns varies dependent on the individual and the type or length of usage of HRT. However, studies to date have shown that the increase in breast density does increase the recall rate in a Breast Screening Service and this may have implications for the future if the use of HRT continues to rise.

Influence on breast cancer risk

With the increase in HRT use concern has been expressed that women using HRT may be at increased risk of developing breast cancer. Recent research indicates that long-term users (more than 8 years) may be at increased risk but that after therapy, the risk returns to normal over time. Further research into the use of HRT and other factors relating to the use of oestrogens will continue.

ANATOMY OF THE ADULT FEMALE BREAST

The external form of the adult female breast varies enormously but its attachment to the chest wall is constant, extending from the fourth to the sixth ribs vertically and from the costal cartilage to the anterior axillary fold transversely. The upper outer quadrant includes a prolongation of breast tissue, known as the axillary tail, which extends towards the axilla. The external rounded form of the breast does not represent the shape of the glandular tissue within the breast. The shape of the breast is due to the fatty tissue which surrounds the glandular elements and which replaces glandular tissue as involution progresses with age. It is the glandular tissue which is essential to demonstrate on a mammogram.

CONGENITAL ANOMALIES

A congenital anomaly occurs when the normal sequence of developmental events takes place in a disordered fashion. Most of the breast anomalies are of academic interest only, but there are a few that are important to a radiographer.

Post- and pre-fixed breasts

In the adult female the developed breast is an approximately hemispherical disc attached by its base to the anterior chest wall and extends from the fourth rib above to the sixth rib below (**Figure 3.8a**). Occasionally the main island of breast tissue happens, by chance, to develop in a position higher (pre-fixed) or lower (post-fixed) than

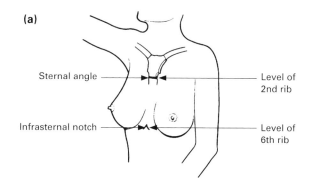

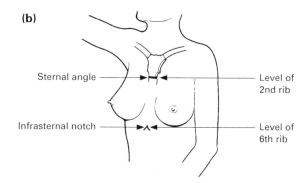

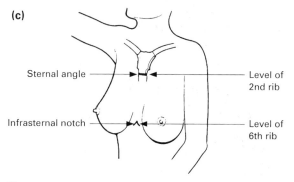

Figure 3.8 Attachment of the breast to the chest wall: (a) usual position (2nd to 6th rib); (b) pre-fixed; (c) post-fixed.

is usual (**Figure 3.8b, c**). In either case the relationship of the breast to the underlying pectoralis muscle will be abnormal and this will be obvious on a medio-lateral oblique mammogram. In a woman with a pre-fixed breast the upper border of the breast can lie as high as the second rib, when its close proximity to the clavicle can make it difficult to achieve satisfactory positioning for adequate mammography. In women with post-fixed breasts the ribs lying above the breast are often clearly evident and the film holder will need to be placed at a lower level than the norm.

Post- and pre-fixed nipples

A breast may be in the normal position on the chest wall but the nipple and areola may develop in an unusually high or low position. This again will be obvious on viewing a medio-lateral oblique mammogram, when there will be an altered relationship between the nipple and the lower corner of the pectoralis shadow. It can be difficult to project pre- and post-fixed nipples in profile, particularly in the cranio-caudal position, and it may be necessary to take a special nipple view.

BREAST CANCER DEVELOPMENT

Breast cancer arises from the epithelial lining of the ducts and lobules. The triggers that create the right environment for the onset of the disease process are not yet fully established but these triggers cause the cells to behave in an aberrant way. Normal cells have a finite life and are replaced by newly developed cells on a regular basis. This is the normal process for cells throughout the body. With breast cancer the cells do not die but continue to thrive and multiply within the confines of the ductal space. Whilst confined to the ductal system the disease, though present, cannot spread.

Once the cancer cells have broken through the basement membrane of the ductal system there is potential for spread into the surrounding breast tissue, the vascular and lymphatic systems and potentially to the rest of the body. Histopathologists apply terms such as minimally invasive, microinvasive to indicate early stages of invasion into the surrounding tissue. Broadly speaking the smaller the invasive component the less likelihood of spread. However, this depends on a multiplicity of factors which lie beyond the remit of this book.

As indicated in subsequent chapters, early stages of breast cancer development can be identified in the majority of cases with mammography. Given some basic understanding of the issue relating to breast cancer development a practitioner in mammography will be fully aware of the potential benefits of mammography to the diagnostic process.

ANATOMICALLY DERIVED MAMMOGRAPHIC PRINCIPLES

- The object of mammography is to demonstrate breast glandular tissue, not fatty tissue or skin. In all projections it is the internal glandular tissue which should be considered and not the outer form of the breast.
- Normal variations on gross anatomy of the breast will influence mammographic technique (**Figure 3.8**)
- Involutionary factors will influence the positioning of the Automatic Exposure Control (**Figure 3.7**)
- It is a fundamental principle of radiography that the x-ray beam is directed at right angles to the longest diameter of the part to be imaged in order to avoid foreshortening. Since it is not the breast fat but the glandular tissue which has to be demonstrated on a mammogram, the longest diameter is that which extends into the upper outer quadrant, at about 45 degrees to the horizontal. It follows that, apart from the medio-lateral oblique, all projections cause foreshortening of the non-involuted gland tissue.
- In all projections the breast should be lifted so that the nipple is level with the centre of the circular attachment of the breast to the chest wall, i.e. to the level of the fourth rib.
- For the medio-oblique projection the film holder angle should be adjusted to reflect the particular stature of the woman. (**Figure 3.6**) Varying the angle to suit the stature of the woman will ensure that:
    - i. the beam is at right angles to the longest diameter of the glandular tissue minimizing foreshortening,
    - iii. compression will be parallel to the correctly positioned pectoralis major thus reducing patient discomfort on compression.

Approximate angles forming the horizontal are as follows:

40 degrees for a short, stocky woman,

45 degrees for the average woman,

50 degrees for a tall woman of slim build.

- Because the breast is attached to a curved chest wall it is inevitable that some breast tissue will be 'cut off' and not be demonstrated on the film

(**see Chapters 5 and 6**). Knowledge of breast development and involutionary processes ensure that any areas excluded will contain fat rather than glandular tissue.

- The comparative mobility of the lateral portions of the breast compared to the medial should be factors considered in mammographic positioning.

FURTHER READING

Beral V, Banks E, Reeves G, Appleby P. Use of HRT and subsequent risk of cancer. *Journal of Epidemiology Biostatistics* 1999; **4** (3): 191–210.

Dixon M. *ABC of Breast Disease 2nd Edition*. London, BMJ Publishing Group, 2000.

Dixon and Sainsbury. *Diseases of the Breast 2nd Edition*. London, Churchill Livingstone, 1998.

Eklund GW, Cardenosa G. The art of mammographic positioning. *Radiological Clinics of North America* 1992; **30** (1): 21–53.

Ellis IO. Terminology of breast disease. *Current Imaging* **1**: 84–90.

Hamilton WJ, Boyd JD, Mossman HW. *Human Embryology*. Cambridge: Heffer, 1949: 323 ff.

Kavanagh AM, Mitchell H, Giles GG. Hormone replacement therapy and accuracy of mammographic screening. *Lancet* 2000; 22: **355** (9200).

Kopans DB. Conventional wisdom: observation, experience, anecdote, and science in breast imaging. *American Journal of Roentgenology* 1994; **162**: 299–303.

Litherland JC, Stallard S, Hole D, Cordiner C. The effect of hormone replacement therapy on the sensitivity of screening mammograms. *Clinical Radiology* 1999; **54**: 285–288.

Lundgren B, Jacobsson S. Single view mammography. *Cancer* 1976; **38**: 1124–1129.

Roebuck EJ. *Clinical Radiology of the Breast*. Oxford: Heinemann Medical Books, 1990: 19–32.

Rutter CM, Mandelson MT, Laya MB, Seger DJ. Changes in breast density associated with initiation, discontinuation, and continuing use of hormone replacement therapy. *JAMA* 2001; **285** (2): 171–176.

Thurjfell EL, Holmberg LH, Persson IR. Screening mammography: sensitivity and specificity in relation to hormone replacement therapy. *Radiology* 1997; **203** (2): 339–341.

Wellings SR. Development of human breast cancer. *Advances in Cancer Research* 1980; **31**: 287–314.

Williams PL, Warwick R, eds. *Gray's Anatomy*. 37th ed. London: Churchill Livingstone, 1989; **156**: 1434–1437.

4

Mammography – the first steps

This chapter provides outlines of:
- importance of clinical background,
- issues of consent and exposure justification,
- communication and the development of a rapport with the patient,
- points of technique relating to all examinations, including anatomical positioning – the 'whole body' technique,
- compression of the breast – why and how.

UNDERSTANDING THE CLINICAL BACKGROUND

Every woman who attends for mammography deserves to be treated as an individual. Women attend a mammography unit for a variety of reasons:

- National or Local Screening Programmes,
- family history surveillance,
- breast symptoms,
- additional views,
- stereotactic-guided needle biopsy and marker localization,
- screening research studies,
- follow-up mammography.

If the woman has been referred for a mammogram because of symptoms, she will be a patient with a problem rather than a well woman, and as such she is more likely to be well motivated. It is likely that she will be tolerant of the procedure, and will probably openly express her anxieties. Amongst these she will already have faced the possibility that her symptoms could be due to cancer. It is more likely that a woman with symptoms will take the opportunity to discuss her problems and anxieties with a mammographer than will a woman attending for screening. The mammographer should be prepared for this, and be prepared to accept the role of sympathetic listener.

In contrast, a woman attending for screening is normally a well woman rather than a patient and she may be unsure of the reason for the invitation to attend the screening clinic. She could be resentful of the procedure, and is likely to expect a higher degree of efficiency, such as the accuracy of time keeping. She may be more anxious about the procedure, and less likely to tolerate discomfort. The possible dangers of radiation may be worrying her and she may well be fearful of the results. Women attending for screening expect a normal outcome while those with symptoms are likely to be better prepared for an abnormal result.

Knowing the reason for attendance can help the mammographer in assessing the client's likely psychological state in relation to the examination. As well as providing essential information, the clinical background will assist in establishing rapport and the validity of the imaging request. *Further information on psychological issues can be obtained in Chapter 13.*

Records of previous attendances will give an insight into any particular difficulties, or the need for a variation of technique. Previous mammograms are of value so that an assessment can be made of unusual mammographic appearances, requiring additional projections or a variation in exposure technique. If forewarned, a mammographer will know what attitude to adopt. In the absence of case notes the mammograms and associated request forms can also give an indication of a woman's previous clinical history.

JUSTIFYING THE EXPOSURE

Recent regulations in Europe have reinforced the essential message that the individual who presses the button (the operator) must be certain that appropriate justification for irradiating the patient has been provided. If requests do not provide sufficient clinical information the radiographer should enquire of the referring clinician.

With reference to age ranges, if a request goes outside the normal protocols and the patents may be at risk from unnecessary radiation, the operator should not proceed until the situation is clarified and the request is justified. A good knowledge and understanding of imaging protocols and, more importantly, the rationale behind them will help the operator make the correct, professional decision thus providing the best care for the mammography client. Students and assistant grade staff will need to refer to the appropriate professional for advice in the first instance.

ISSUES OF INFORMED OR VALID CONSENT

It is not the purpose of this book to set out the legal debate on consent as this will vary from country to country, state to state, and hospital to hospital. However, every professional should ensure that they have an understanding of these issues and the local approach to this. It is essential that the mammographer is sure that the woman attending has enough knowledge on which to proceed with the examination.

In the screening situation the issue of consent is complex. Women attending for screening need to know that the test is not 100% effective and that a recall for further tests is a possibility before proceeding with the examination. It could be suggested that women attending with symptoms are more consenting to mammography: nevertheless, the patient's choice to proceed or otherwise must always be respected. In all cases the mammographer needs to recognize when the woman who has arrived willingly, later withdraws consent at some point during the procedure.

A further issue of informed consent relates to those who are brought to the unit by relatives or professional care staff. There has been a general thrust to bring all eligible women to screening centres thus providing equal access for all. However, patients in this group can be assisted to understand the process with the use of appropriate guidance. This can be in the form of images, sign language, demonstration and through the relative or carer. It should be noted that the client has the final choice and the mammographer needs to be sensitive to the client's wishes, however these are demonstrated.

PRE-MAMMOGRAPHY DISCUSSION

Establishing rapport

Communication skills are important in the radiographer–patient relationship. This is never more true than in mammography. A woman's perception of a mammographic service largely depends on the performance and communication skills of the mammography practitioner. The opportunity for the mammographer to communicate with a woman should be scheduled into the appointment times. A patient's anxiety will be significantly increased if insufficient time is available for her and the practitioner to communicate.

Immediately before the examination is the best opportunity to build up a rapport with a woman and help her to feel comfortable about the examination. Having a physically relaxed woman is an essential prerequisite to obtaining high-quality mammography. Any questions the woman raises should be answered frankly and openly. If a mammographer does not know the answer he/she should say so and suggest a likely source for the information. It is important that the mammographer should not give reassurance beyond his/her own field of competence.

Explaining the procedure

Some time should be spent with the woman explaining the examination. A woman attending for the first time is highly likely to have heard an inaccurate account of the mammographic examination from friends or neighbours. They could have told her that to have a mammogram is very uncomfortable, possibly that it is agony. In order to obtain maximal co-operation, these fears should be countered with a clear concise explanation of exactly what the examination entails. Phrases to use during the explanation might include comments such as:

- 'it is uncomfortable rather than painful',
- 'if it does become too uncomfortable, don't hesitate to tell me',

- 'it doesn't last long – only a few seconds for each film',
- 'compression is essential to obtain good pictures and to show details clearly',
- 'the pressure will not harm your breasts'.

Relevant history

In many units it is the usual practice for the mammographer to take a brief medical history before the examination. This is useful both in establishing patient rapport and in obtaining information about relevant breast symptoms that could assist in the later interpretation of the mammograms by the radiologist. Details worth recording include:

- A brief summary of the reason for the current examination.
- Past history of breast disease, the suspected diagnosis at the time and any treatment given, especially the site and date of any previous surgery.
- Details of any scars or skin lesions should be marked on a diagram.
- Any reported breast symptom.
- Some centres feel it is appropriate to record any history of breast cancer in the family.
- In some centres a note is also made of any hormone replacement therapy, including duration and type of treatment.

Observing and reporting clinical signs

All clients attending for symptomatic clinics will have perceived symptoms, however, some women in screening attend with symptoms also. It is important to note these symptoms and indicate to those reading the films of the patients concerns. It is also important for the mammographer to note details of any significant clinical signs she or he may observe during the procedure. These signs may indicate an underlying abnormality which may not be demonstrated on mammography and could bring to the attention of the team an occult breast cancer. Important signs to note include:

- a lump,
- skin tethering or dimpling,
- recent nipple inversion,
- eczema of the nipple,
- nipple discharge.

All mammographers are recommended to spend some time in a breast clinic with a specialist clinician, observing examination of women with symptoms so that skills in recognizing significant clinical signs of breast disease are acquired.

IMPORTANT POINTS OF TECHNIQUE

There are some points of technique that apply to all mammographic projections, and that should be regarded as 'golden rules'. The following notes outline the more important of these.

Film marking

To assist in orientation, annotations should always be placed on the lateral/axillary edge and at the corner of the film away from the woman. Care should be taken to check the identity of the client, and to make sure that all information put on the film is correct.

Anatomical positioning

From the point of view of patient positioning, mammography is a whole body technique. The correct positioning of the woman's feet, arms and spine are important in obtaining high-quality diagnostic mammograms. It is essential, therefore, to consider all these aspects of patient positioning throughout the examination. The position of the woman's whole body must be manipulated and controlled by the radiographer for the breast to be examined properly. This task is most easily achieved by performing the examination with the woman standing.

On occasions a woman may have to be examined while she is seated and it is perfectly possible to achieve excellent mammograms in this position. Specially designed examination chairs with full and adjustable lumbar support make this task much simpler for the woman and the examining radiographer. The chair should be on wheels with an easily operated, foot-activated braking system.

Manipulating and controlling the breast

Handling the breast can be difficult for the practitioner, particularly in early stages of training. The breast should be held firmly, the hand cupping the breast with the thumb and fingers at the posterior margin of the breast against the chest wall; the internal structures of the breast must be grasped, not just the overlying fat. Handling the breast in this manner will maintain control of the breast throughout the procedure and ensure the patient has confidence in the radiographer.

COMPRESSION OF THE BREAST

Compression of the breast tissue is essential for good mammography (**Table 4.1**). Before an examination the woman should be clearly and simply told about the need for breast compression. It is then less likely that she will find the examination uncomfortable.

When applying compression, control of the whole woman should be maintained, as detailed above, with one hand controlling the position of the woman's body while the other manipulates the breast. As the compression plate descends onto the breast and begins to hold it firmly the hand controlling the breast should be moved forward slowly from the chest wall towards the nipple. Care should be taken to ensure that the hand does not itself take any of the compression

Table 4.1 Beneficial effects of breast compression during mammography

Reduction of internal x-ray beam scatter
Improved contrast
Spreading of breast tissues:
    reduced superimposition
    clearer demonstration
Reduced geometric unsharpness
Reduced movement unsharpness
Reduced radiation dose to the breast
More homogeneous film density

force. There is considerable skill involved in applying compression without losing control of the breast position; the novice will almost certainly experience some difficulties with this initially.

In the past, mammographers were encouraged to apply as much compression force as possible to the breast. Standard teaching was 'not moderate compression, but the most vigorous possible compression tolerated by the patient'. One reason for this advice was that, at the time when this technique was being recommended, it was standard practice to place the corner of the film high in the axilla. This resulted in compression being applied to the anterior axillary fold in addition to the breast itself. The firmness of the anterior axillary fold made it difficult to apply sufficient compression to the breast itself. This meant that a greater degree of force was required to overcome the resistance of the axillary fold tissue. Much of the resultant pain originated from compression of the axillary muscles and overlying soft tissues.

Modern mammographic technique (see **Chapter 5**) requires the breast to be placed centrally on the film with compression applied to breast tissue and not the axillary fold. This technique ensures better demonstration of the breast itself at the expense of imaging the armpit, but is much less likely to cause pain.

There is an optimum level of compression beyond which extra force ceases to have any perceptible effect on image quality or any significant reduction in radiation dose. However, the additional force does have a marked effect on the woman's tolerance of the procedure. 'Discomfort' becomes 'pain' if that 'little bit more' compression is applied.

In the United Kingdom the maximum force permitted to be applied to the breast is 200 Newtons. The majority of recently produced machines have a limiting level of approximately 160 Newtons. In normal practice this amount of force should not be necessary. A local survey of experienced radiographers found that excellent quality mammograms were consistently achieved by applying a maximum force of 140 Newtons (**Table 4.2**).

Table 4.2 Range of force (newtons) applied to the breast during the production of good-quality mammograms

Projection	Range of forces used (newtons)
Craniocaudal	70–140
Mediolateral oblique	100–140
Lateral	70–140

REFERENCES AND FURTHER READING

Dixon M. *ABC of Breast Disease 2nd Edition*. London, BMJ Publishing Group, 2000.

Dixon JM, Sainsbury JRC. *Handbook of Diseases of the Breast 2nd Edition*. London, Churchill Livingstone, 1998.

Ekland GW. Mammography compression: science or art? *Radiology* 1991; **181**: 339–341.

Ellman R, Angeli N, Christians A, Moss S, Chamberlain J, Maguire PP. Psychiatric morbidity associated with screening for breast cancer. *British Journal Cancer* 1989; **60**: 781–784.

Fentimann I, Hisham H. *Atlas of Breast Examination*. London, BMJ Publishing Group.

Logan WW, Norlund AW. Screen/film mammography technique: compression and other factors. In: Logan WW, ed. *Reduced Dose Mammography*. New York: Masson Publishing, 1979; 415–428.

Lovegrove M. Results of a survey carried out amongst radiographers in NHSBSP. *Proceedings of Symposium Mammographicum*, London, 1992.

Puolos A, Rickard M. Compression in mammography and the perception of discomfort. *Australasian Radiology* 1997; **41** (3): 247–252.

Nielsen B. Technical aspects of mammography. *Current Opinion in Radiology* 1992; **4**: 118–122.

Rickards MT. *Mammography Today for Radiographers*. Sydney: Central Sydney X-ray Programme, 1992.

Roebuck EJ. *Clinical Radiology of the Breast*. Oxford: Heinemann, 1990: 60 pp.

Rutter DR, Calnan M, Valie MSB, Wade CA. Discomfort and pain during mammography. Description, prediction and prevention. *British Medical Journal* 1992; **304**: 22.

Sardenelli F, Zandrino F, Imperiale A, Bonaldo E, Qaurtini MG, Cogorno N. Breast biphasic compression versus standard monophasic compression in x-ray mammography. *Radiology* 2000; **217**: 576–580.

5

Mammography – basic projections

This chapter provides outlines of:

- how to perform the basic mammographic projections
  (a) the routine cranio-caudal
  (b) the 45 degree medio-lateral oblique,
- how to recognize and rectify positioning faults as they arise,
- how to recognize the adequacy of the examination.

THE CRANIO-CAUDAL PROJECTION

Indications

The cranio-caudal projection combined with the 45 degree medio-lateral oblique mammogram is the routine for all initial x-ray examinations of the breast.

Area demonstrated

The majority of breast tissue is demonstrated with the exclusion of the extreme medial portion and the axillary tail (**Figures 5.1** and **5.2**).

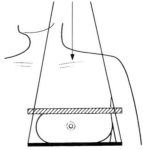

Figure 5.1   The cranio-caudal projection.

31

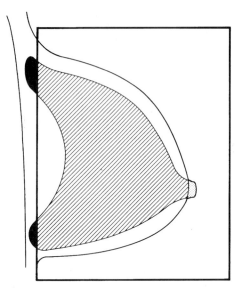

Figure 5.2   The area demonstrated.

Equipment position

The breast support table is horizontal and raised to slightly above the level of inframammary angle.

Anatomical position – left breast
(Figure 5.3)

The woman faces the machine, about 5–6 cm back, with her feet pointing towards the

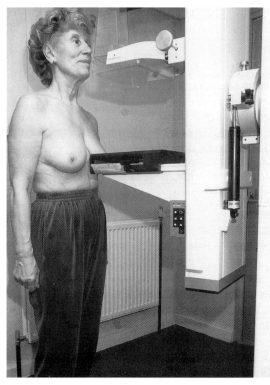

Figure 5.3

machine. Her arms are by her side. The breast to be examined should be aligned with the centre of the table. The mammographer should stand medial of the breast to be examined.

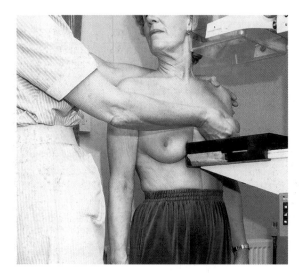

Figure 5.4

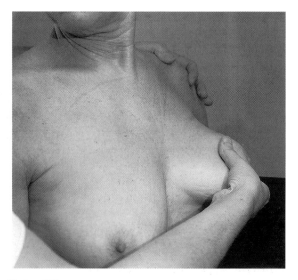

Figure 5.5

Breast positioning (Figure 5.4, 5.5)

1.

- Lift the left breast up and away from the chest wall with your right hand.
- Hold the woman's left shoulder with your left hand.
- Turn her head to the right.

Alternative technique for the radiographer of short stature

1a.

- Lift the left breast up and away from the chest wall with your right hand.
- Place your left hand on the left scapula (**Figure 5.6**).
- Turn the woman's head to the right.

2. Encourage her to lean forward, rotating the thorax a few degrees to bring the rib cage directly below the nipple line against the edge of the breast support table (**Figure 5.7**).

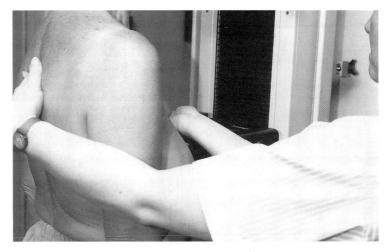

Figure 5.6

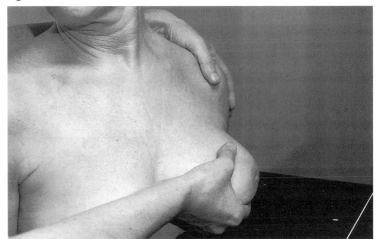

Figure 5.7

3. Keep hold of her left shoulder and remove your hand from beneath the breast so that the breast rests on the support table (**Figure 5.8**). **Using the light beam diaphragm, check that:**

a. the nipple is in profile,
b. the medial portion of the breast is on the film,
c. the shoulder is relaxed in order that the upper lateral portion of the breast is on the film,
d. the image field covers all the tissue in front of the thorax.

If the criteria are not achieved refer to **Table 5.1**.

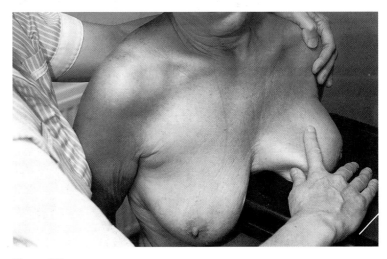

Figure 5.8

Table 5.1 Trouble shooting

Problem	Cause	Corrective action
Nipple pointing downwards	The film holder is too high	Decrease the height of the film holder
	The skin on the underside of the breast is caught at the edge of the film holder	Lift the breast again, pulling forward the underside of the breast
	Excess loose skin on the superior surface of the breast	Control the nipple position by gently applying tension to the skin surface as compression is applied. N.B. Move only the skin surface, not the underlying tissue
	The woman has a post-fixed nipple	No improvement can be made without loss of breast tissue
		Either take a supplementary view and/or ensure a clear view of the retro-areolar region on the medio-lateral oblique
Folds at the lateral aspect	Pad of fat/skin above upper outer quadrant	Alter the position of the arm: 1. Put her hand on her hip 2. Put the palm of her hand on her abdomen 3. Put her hand on her shoulder with her elbow back 4. Bring her hand forward beneath support table to hold on at the far side
	The woman is leaning towards the medial	Lift the breast, encourage her to step a little to the medial and lean to the lateral
	The breast is twisted	Using the thumb and third finger of your right hand lift the breast and push the superior surface laterally and pull the inferior surface medially

Applying the compression

1. Hold the left shoulder with your left hand, exerting gentle pressure downwards. Place your right thumb on the medial aspect of the breast and the first two fingers of your right hand on the superior surface, pulling gently forward towards the nipple (**Figure 5.9**).

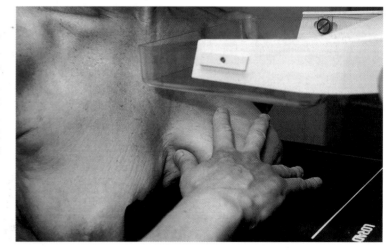

Figure 5.9

2. Using the foot pedal, apply compression slowly and evenly, gradually moving your hand towards the nipple until the hand is replaced by the compression plate (**Figure 5.10**).

Remember:

- Control the body and the breast until compression is complete.
- Expose immediately.
- Release compression as soon as exposure has terminated.

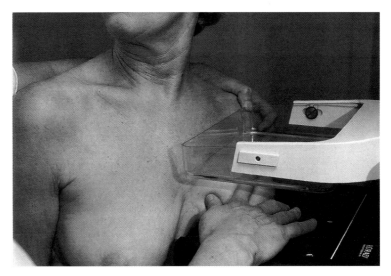

Figure 5.10

The cranio-caudal should demonstrate:

- the nipple in profile and pointing towards the centre of the long axis of the film,
- the majority of medial tissue,
- the majority of the lateral tissue with the exclusion of the axillary tail,
- pectoral muscle demonstrated at the centre of the film on approximately 30% of individuals,
- the depth of breast tissue demonstrated should be equal to, or no more than 1 cm less than, the distance from the nipple to pectoral muscle on the medio-lateral oblique projection.

The breast in the cranio-caudal position is shown in **Figure 5.11** and the resulting mammogram in **Figure 5.12**.

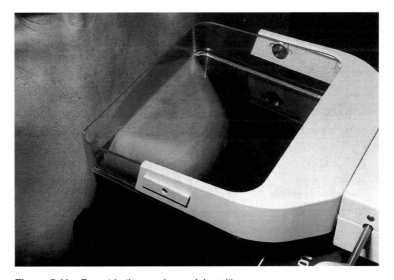

Figure 5.11   Breast in the cranio-caudal position.

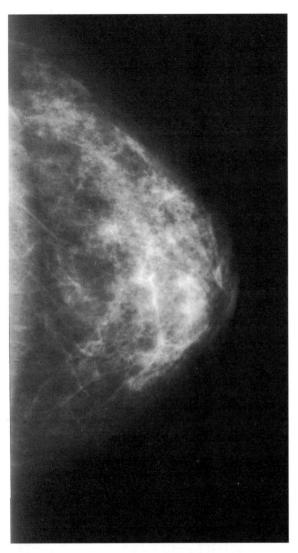

Figure 5.12 The cranio-caudal mammogram.

THE 45 DEGREE MEDIO-LATERAL OBLIQUE PROJECTION

The technique described below is a structured approach to the oblique projection which breaks down each movement in order that the student of mammography is able to maximize the chances of producing a high-quality mammogram.

The advantages of the method described are:

- The demonstration of the inframammary angle, frequently an area of difficulty for the mammographer is given high priority.
- Skin folds in the axillary region are eliminated.
- The complex movement required to place the axilla accurately can be fully explained to the trainee mammographer.

Indications

The medio-lateral oblique projection (**Figure 5.13**) is used in all routine mammographic examinations together with the cranio-caudal projection.

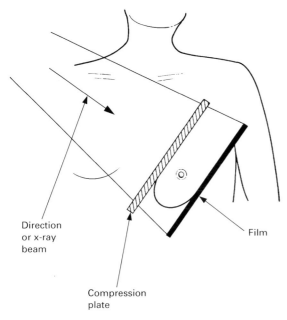

Figure 5.13 The 45 degree medio-lateral oblique projection.

Area demonstrated

Carefully performed, the lateral oblique mammogram is the only projection in which all the breast tissue can be demonstrated on one film (**Figure 5.14**).

Equipment position

The machine should be rotated through 45 degrees. The top of the breast support table should be level with the notch beneath the clavicle and humeral head when the woman's arm is by her side.

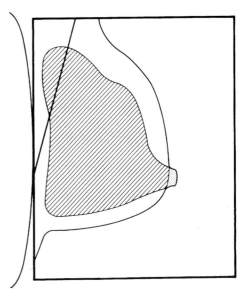

Figure 5.14   The area demonstrated.

Anatomical position – left breast
(Figure 5.15)

The woman faces the machine with her feet pointing towards the machine. The lateral edge of the thorax should be in line with the edge of the breast support table. The radiographer should stand slightly behind and to the right of the woman.

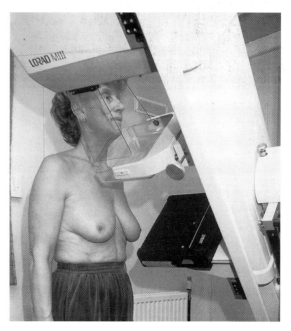

Figure 5.15

Breast positioning

1. Ask the woman to place her left hand on her head and lift her chin up. Hold the left breast in your right hand. Hold the left shoulder in your left hand (**Figure 5.16, 5.17**).

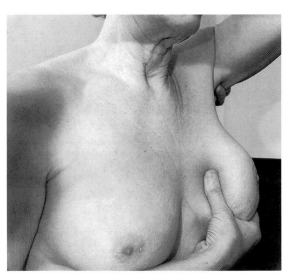

Figure 5.17

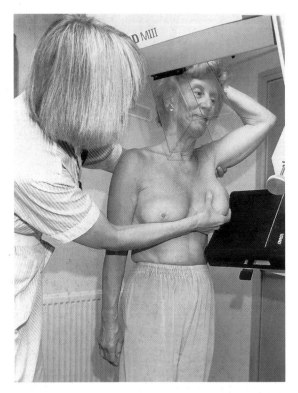

Figure 5.16

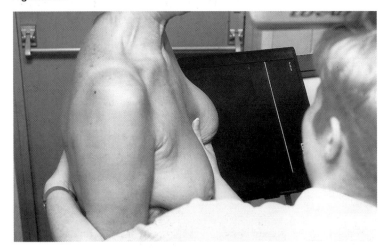

Figure 5.18

Alternative positioning for the radiographer of small stature

1a.

- Place the left hand on the scapula instead of the humeral head.
- Lift the breast up and away from the chest wall with your right hand so that the whole breast is supported and the nipple profile can be seen (**Figure 5.18**).

2. **Keeping the nipple in profile**, encourage her to lean forward into the machine, and then slightly laterally (**Figure 5.19**). Using the light beam diaphragm check that:

   (a) the nipple is still in profile,

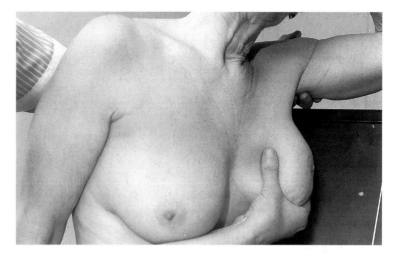

Figure 5.19

   (b) the inframammary angle is within the radiation field (**Figure 5.20**).

If the criteria are not met refer to **Table 5.2**.

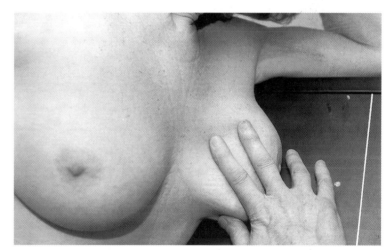

Figure 5.20

Table 5.2   Trouble shooting

Problem	Cause	Corrective action
Nipple rotated towards breast support table	The woman's skin is caught on the table at the lateral aspect	Lift the breast again and pull through at the lateral edge
Nipple rotated towards the tube	The hips and/or feet are rotated	Straighten the hips and feet so that they are pointing towards the machine
Inframammary angle not visualized	The hips and/or feet are rotated	Straighten the hips and feet so that they are pointing towards the machine
	The woman is standing too far behind the table	Encourage her to step 6–8 cm towards you

3. When the nipple is in profile and the inframammary angle clearly demonstrated, go behind the breast support table, ensuring that the woman keeps her thorax in the same position.
4. Ask the woman to remove her hand from her head. Take her left wrist in your left hand. Place your right hand on her left shoulder, lifting the posterior skin edge of the axilla with your thumb (**Figure 5.21**).

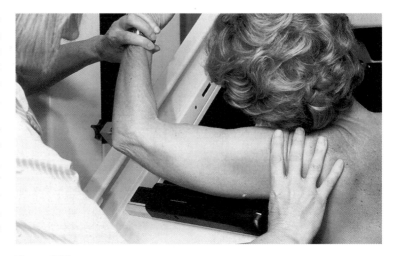

Figure 5.21

5. Gently pull her arm across the corner of, and behind, the support table at an angle of approximately 45 degrees (**Figure 5.22**). At the same time, encourage her to rotate the humeral head forward with the palm of your right hand.
6. Bring the woman's arm down, bending it so that she can rest her right hand on the machine handle in a comfortable position with the elbow hanging down behind the support table (**Figure 5.23**). Ensure that the corner of the support table lies in the axilla, immediately anterior to the posterior axillary fold.

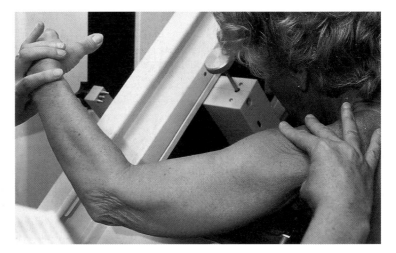

Figure 5.22

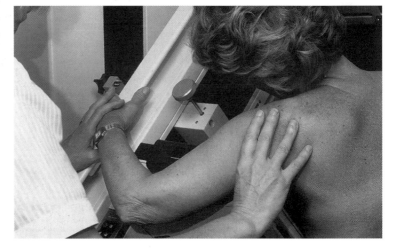

Figure 5.23

Alternative technique for the radiographer of short stature

3a. Ask the woman to place her left hand on the handle bar (**Figure 5.24**).

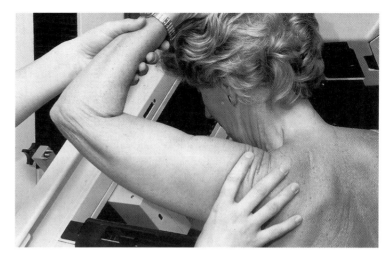

Figure 5.24

4a. Hold the left elbow with your left hand, place your right hand on her left shoulder, lifting the posterior skin edge of the axilla with your thumb. Lift the elbow to rotate the humeral head anteriorly, pull her arm across and behind the top of the film holder at approximately 45 degrees (**Figure 5.25**).

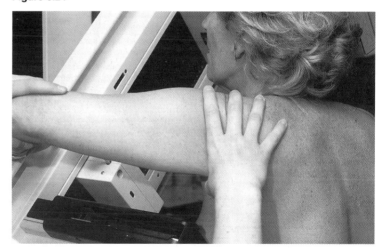

Figure 5.25

5a. Place the axilla on the corner of the support table ensuring that the table lies immediately anterior to the posterior axillary fold (**Figure 5.26**).

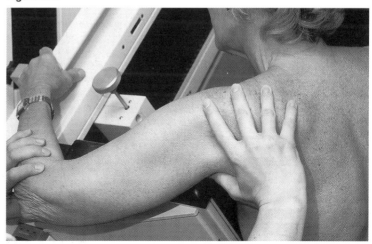

Figure 5.26

6a. Release the elbow, allowing it to hang down comfortably behind the support table (**Figure 5.27**).

Remember:

- The left hand controls the arm movement.
- The right hand controls the shoulder and humeral head.
- The right thumb lifts the posterior flap of the axilla until the shoulder is in place on the corner of the table.

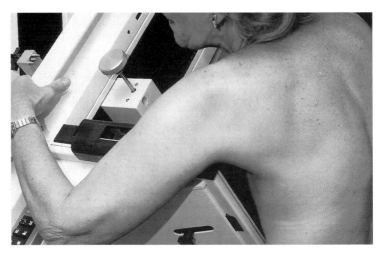

Figure 5.27

7. Ensuring that the woman does not move, return to the front of the support table. Use the right hand to check for creases in the axilla and at the lateral aspect (**Figure 5.28**).

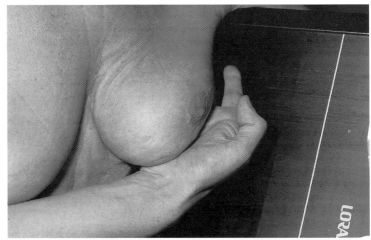

Figure 5.28

8. Check for potential creases at the inframammary angle (**Figure 5.29**).

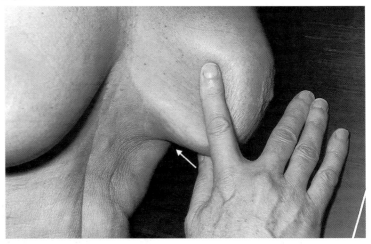

Figure 5.29

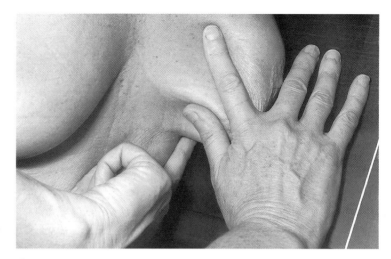

9. Tidy the inframammary angle (**Figure 5.30–5.32**).

Figure 5.30

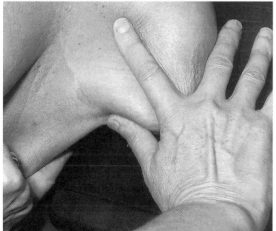

Figure 5.31

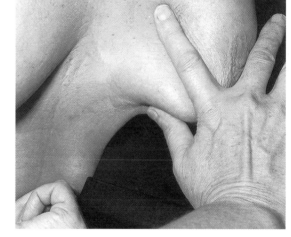

Figure 5.32

10. Before applying compression, use the light beam diaphragm to check (**Figure 5.33**) that:
    a. the pectoral muscle is across the film by ensuring that the compression plate will be adjacent to the thorax from immediately beneath the clavicle to the inframammary angle,
    b. the nipple is in profile,
    c. the inframammary angle is clearly visible,
    d. there are no skin folds.

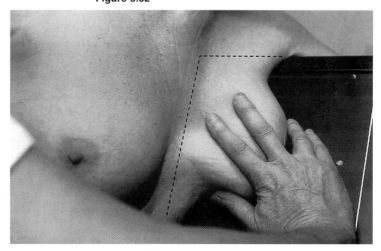

Figure 5.33

If criteria are not met, refer to **Table 5.3**.

Table 5.3 Trouble shooting

Problem	Cause	Corrective action
Pectoral muscle not across the film	The film may be too high	Reduce height of machine 2–3 cm Pull arm across film again and re-settle shoulder
Nipple no longer in profile and/or inframammary angle no longer demonstrated	The pectoral muscle has been taken too far across the film, with the result that the woman has rotated her thorax and/or hips	Re-adjust shoulder position so that the thorax and hips can be turned back into position
	The film may be too high and the breast is taut	Lower the film so that the breast is relaxed
Folds at the inframammary angle	Overlap of lower border of breast and abdominal wall. Compression will exaggerate this and push the inframammary angle off the film	Insert forefinger between support table and the lateral edge of the breast. Hook out surplus tissue and pull down and tuck behind film holder (see **Figures 5.30, 5.31, 5.32**)
Folds across the axilla (rings of Saturn)	The film may be too high so that excessive lift of the breast creates a crease	Lower the film by 2–3 cm with the woman still in position
	The woman has large breasts with a pad of fat/breast tissue in the axillary tail	1. Attempt to smooth out the skin surface as compression is applied, placing a finger at the lateral aspect of the breast and sweeping the skin surface upwards 2. Two views may be necessary (see **Chapter 6**)

Applying compression

1. Hold the woman's left shoulder in the left hand. Lift the left breast, with the right hand, up and away from the chest wall. Maintaining the lift on the medial aspect of the breast, spread the fingers across the breast ready to apply compression (**Figure 5.34**).

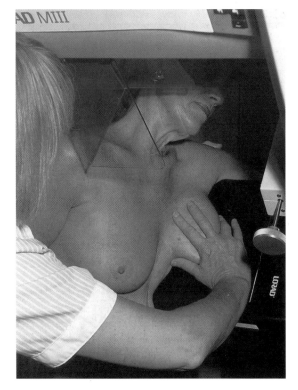

Figure 5.34

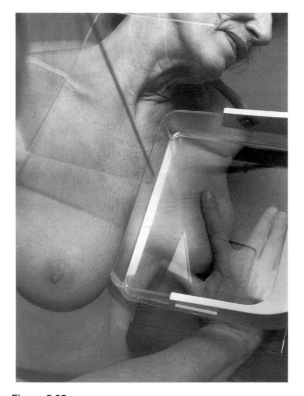

Figure 5.35

2. Using the foot pedal, apply compression evenly and slowly, gradually moving the fingers forward, towards the nipple, maintaining lift with your thumb until the compression plate has taken firm hold of the breast (**Figure 5.35**).

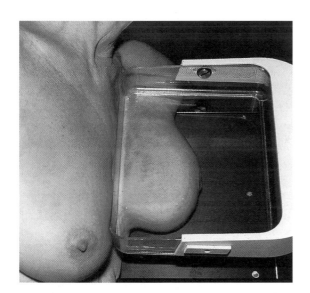

Figure 5.36 Breast in the 45 degree medio-lateral oblique position.

Remember:

- The left hand controls the body.
- The right hand controls the breast.
- Expose immediately.
- Release compression after exposure.

The 45 degree medio-lateral oblique mammogram should demonstrate:

- the inframammary angle,
- the nipple in profile,
- the nipple lifted to the level of the lower border of the pectoral muscle,
- the pectoral muscle across the film at an appropriate angle for the individual woman (generally between 20 and 35 degrees from the vertical).

The final position is shown in **Figure 5.36** and the resultant mammogram in **Figure 5.37**.

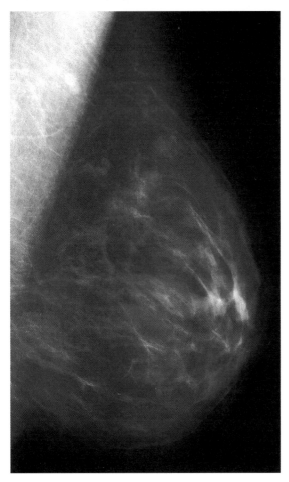

Figure 5.37 The 45 degree medio-lateral oblique mammogram.

Difficulties with even application of compression

It is not infrequent for novice mammographers to experience difficulties with applying compression. The compression paddle holds the axilla but the breast itself droops. This is a result of 'bulk' at the axilla and frequently occurs with heavily built women.

In order to reduce this bulk the axillary region should be repositioned so that the elbow hangs down behind the film holder and the pectoral muscle is brought parallel to the film. If the problem continues the film should be slightly lowered and the procedure repeated.

In severe cases, when women have large breasts, as well as being heavily built, two views may be necessary (see **Chapter 7**).

Adjusting to the individual

In order to facilitate accurate positioning in the medio-lateral oblique position, consideration of the woman's anatomy must be taken. The reasons behind this are fully explained in **Chapter 3**.

However, as a general rule, if a woman has narrow shoulders with small breasts a slightly steeper angle of 50–55 degrees from the horizontal should be selected, if accurate positioning proves difficult.

In the case of a woman with broad shoulders, a flatter angle of 40 degrees from the horizontal may prove more successful.

FURTHER READING

Andolina VF, Lille SL, Willison KM. *Mammography Imaging: a Practical Guide*. Philadelphia: JB Lippincott, 1992.
Bassett LW, Hirbawi IA, DeBruhl N, Hayes MK. Mammographic positioning: evaluation from the view box. *Radiology* 1993; **188** (3): 803–806.
Ekland GW. Mammography compression: science or art? *Radiology* 1991; **181**: 339–341.
Logan WW, Janus J. Use of special mammographic views to maximize radiographic information. *Radiological Clinics of North America* 1987; **25**: 953–959.
Lundgren B, Jacobson S. Single view mammography. *Cancer* 1976; **38**: 1124–1129.
Naylor SM, York J. An evaluation of the pectoral muscle to nipple level as a component to assess the quality of the medio-lateral oblique mammogram. *Radiography* 1999; **5**: 107–110.

Naylor S, Lee L, Evans A. A study to find the optimal orientation of the cranio-caudal view for screening purposes. *Clinical Radiology* 1999; **54**: 804–806.
NHSBSP. *Quality Assurance Guidelines for Radiographers*. National Health Service Breast Screening Programme Publication No. 30. Sheffield: NHSBSP Publications, 1994.
Rickards MT. *Mammography Today for Radiographers*. Sydney: Central Sydney X-ray Programme, 1992.
Sickles EA. Practical solutions to common mammographic problems: tailoring the examination. *American Journal of Roentgenology* 1988; **151**: 31–39.
Wentz G. *Mammography for Radiologic Technologists*. New York: McGraw Hill, 1992.

6

Mammography – complementary projections

This chapter outlines how to:

- perform additional mammographic projections which may be required for assessment of a possible abnormality in the breast,
- evaluate the accuracy of positioning,
- localize lesions accurately for special procedures,
- image specimens of core-cut, Mammotome and excision biopsies.

MEDIALLY ROTATED CRANIO-CAUDAL PROJECTION

Indications

This projection is indicated for:

- lesions demonstrated in the medio-lateral oblique but not on the cranio-caudal projection,
- lesions located in the extreme lateral portion of the breast,
- large breasted women who require more than one film in the cranio-caudal position.

Area demonstrated

This projection shows the lateral and mid-line portions of the breast (**Figure 6.1** and **6.2**).

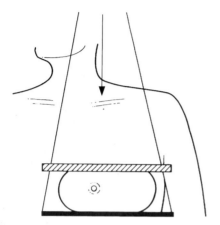

Figure 6.1 The medially rotated cranio-caudal projection.

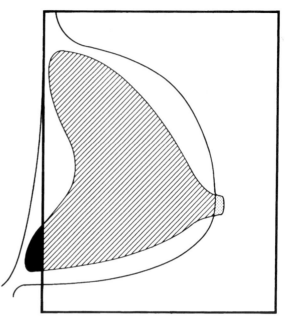

Figure 6.2 The area demonstrated.

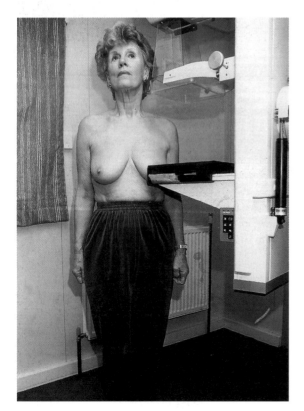

Figure 6.3

Equipment position

The breast support table is horizontal and raised to just above the level of the inframammary angle.

Anatomical position – left breast

The woman faces the machine, about 5–6 cm back, with the feet turned 5–10 degrees to the right. The breast should be aligned slightly to the right of centre of the table. Her head should be turned to the right (**Figure 6.3**).

Breast positioning

1. Lift the left breast with the right hand. Hold the left shoulder with your left hand (**Figure 6.4**).

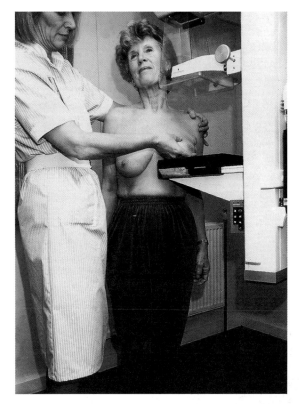

Figure 6.4

2. Encourage the woman to lean into the machine, bringing the lateral portion of the breast on to the film. The medial portion of the breast will not be on the film. Her shoulder should be relaxed. Ensure the nipple is in profile and that there are no skin folds on the superior and inferior skin surfaces (**Figure 6.5**).

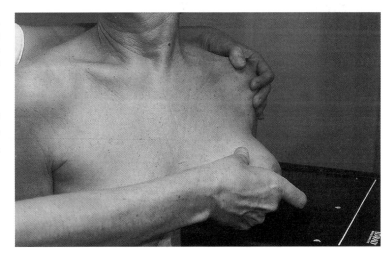

Figure 6.5

3. Hold the left breast with your right hand and her left shoulder with your left hand (**Figure 6.6**). Maintaining the forward pull on the lateral aspect of the breast, apply compression using the compression plate to enhance this effect. Expose immediately and release.

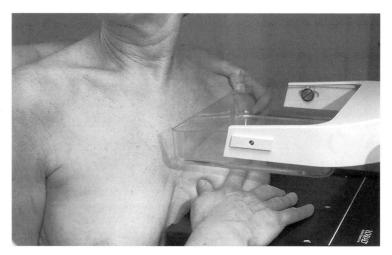

Figure 6.6

The final medially rotated cranio-caudal position and resultant mammogram are illustrated in **Figures 6.7** and **6.8**:

- the nipple points towards the medial,
- the muscle may be demonstrated, in the lateral portion of the breast.

Difficulties with the medially rotated cranio-caudal projection

The head of the humerus may prevent clear imaging of the lateral aspect on some women. A suitable alternative would be the extended cranio-caudal.

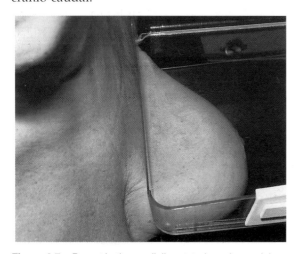

Figure 6.7   Breast in the medially rotated cranio-caudal position.

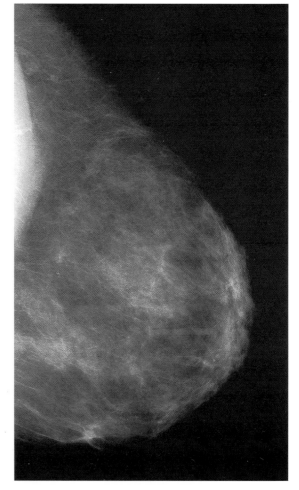

Figure 6.8   The medially rotated mammogram.

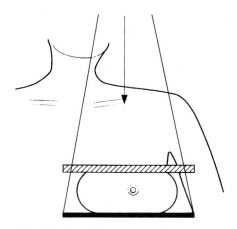

Figure 6.9   The laterally rotated cranio-caudal projection.

LATERALLY ROTATED CRANIO-CAUDAL PROJECTION

Indications

Occasionally a lesion may be demonstrated on the medio-lateral oblique which is not evident on the standard cranio-caudal view. If the whole lateral aspect has been demonstrated on this view it is a possibility that the lesion lies medially.

Area demonstrated

The extreme medial portion of breast and the skin over the sternum are shown (**Figures 6.9, 6.10**).

Equipment position

The breast support table is horizontal and raised to just above the level of the inframammary angle.

Anatomical position – left breast

The woman faces the machine, with her feet straight on, and her body as close as possible to the table. The breast should be aligned slightly right of centre of the support table (**Figure 6.11**).

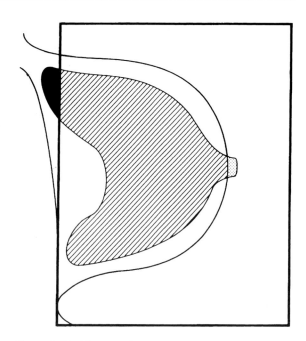

Figure 6.10   The area demonstrated.

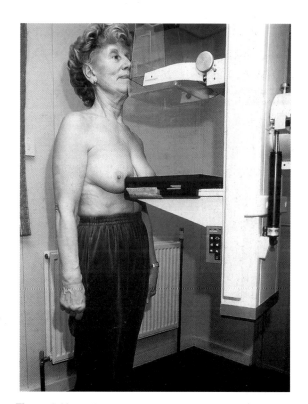

Figure 6.11

Breast positioning

1. Hold the left breast with your right hand and place your left hand on the mid-dorsal region (**Figure 6.12**).

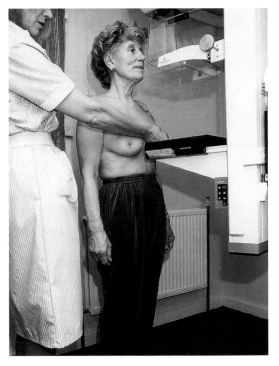

Figure 6.12

2. Lift the left breast onto the support table, bringing the medial portion of the breast onto the film (**Figure 6.13**).

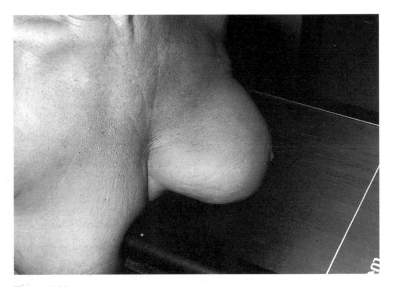

Figure 6.13

3. Lift the medial portion of the **RIGHT** breast on to the film to prevent drag on the left breast and to aid demonstration of the cleavage (**Figure 6.14**).

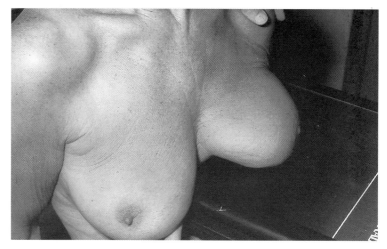

Figure 6.14

4. Encourage the woman to lean forward and medially so that her head is at the side of the tube housing (**Figure 6.15**).

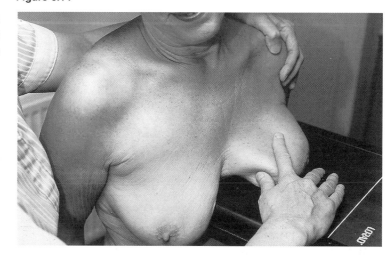

Figure 6.15

5. Ensure that the medial portions of both breasts are pulled forward and fold free and that the sternum is against the support table. Put your left hand on the mid-dorsal area to maintain forward pressure (**Figure 6.16**). Pulling the medial portion of the left breast forward with the right hand, apply compression using the compression plate to enhance the pull forward on the medial breast tissue. Expose immediately and release.

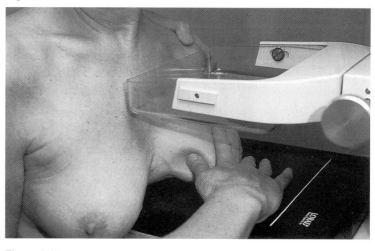

Figure 6.16

The final laterally rotated cranio-caudal position and resultant mammogram are illustrated in **Figure 6.17** and **6.18**:

- the nipple points towards the lateral,
- the cleavage may be demonstrated.

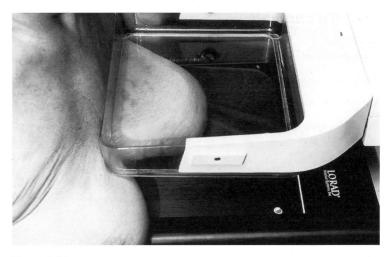

Figure 6.17

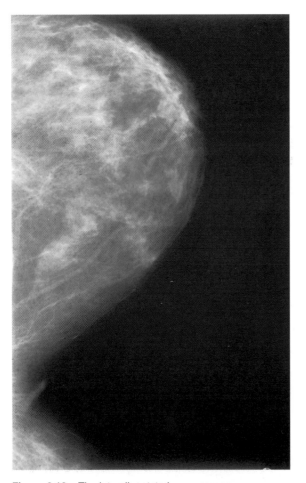

Figure 6.18   The laterally rotated mammogram.

Difficulties encountered

Imaging the medial portion of the breast can be difficult for the woman, as the tube housing may be in the way of her head. Frequent encouragement is required to optimize imaging.

EXTENDED CRANIO-CAUDAL PROJECTION

Indications

This projection is used to show a lesion seen high in the axillary tail on the medio-lateral oblique but not demonstrated on a cranio-caudal.

Area demonstrated

The axillary tail and upper midline portion of breast tissue are demonstrated (**Figures 6.19, 6.20**).

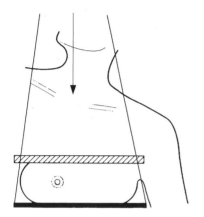

Figure 6.19 The extended cranio-caudal projection.

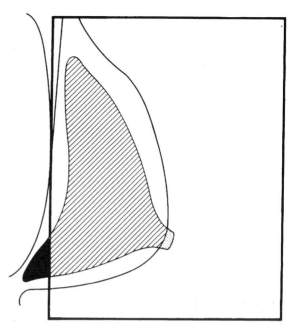

Figure 6.20 The area demonstrated.

Equipment position

The machine should be raised some 5–10 degrees from the horizontal at the lateral aspect. It should be slightly below the level of the inframammary angle (**Figure 6.21**).

Anatomical position – left breast

The woman should stand close to the machine with her breast aligned slightly right of centre of the table and her feet and hips pointing towards the machine.

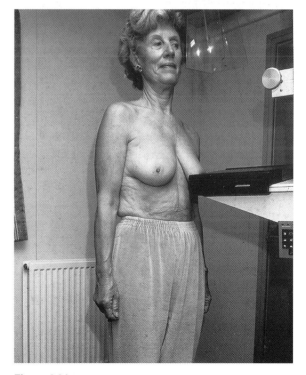

Figure 6.21

Breast positioning

1. Hold the left breast in your right hand and the shoulder in your left (**Figure 6.22**).

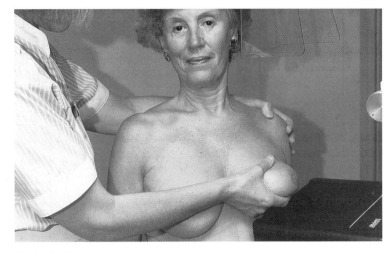

Figure 6.22

2. Lift the breast up and place on the film holder (**Figure 6.23**).

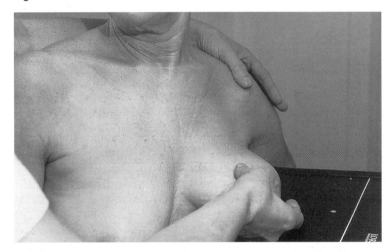

Figure 6.23

3. Encourage the woman to lean some 10–15 degrees to the lateral, extending her arm away from the side of her body (**Figure 6.24**). The woman must remain facing the machine directly, and should not rotate her thorax into an oblique position. Apply compression, expose and release immediately.

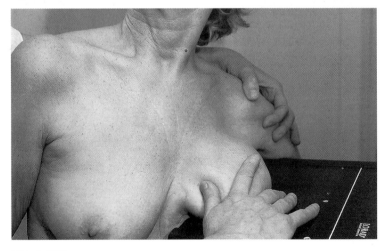

Figure 6.24

The final extended cranio-caudal position and resultant mammogram are illustrated in **Figures 6.25** and **6.26**.

The extended cranio-caudal projection should demonstrate:

- the nipple in profile,
- the anterior edge of the pectoral muscle lateral to the midline of the breast.

Difficulties encountered

This is an awkward position for the woman, and compression, exposure and release should be accomplished with speed.

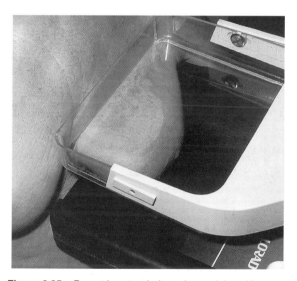

Figure 6.25   Breast in extended cranio-caudal position.

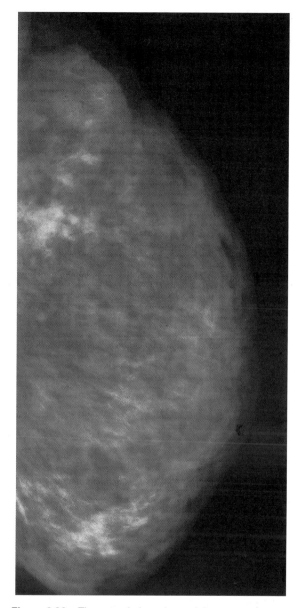

Figure 6.26   The extended cranio-caudal mammogram.

MEDIO-LATERAL PROJECTION

Indications

This projection is indicated for the following:

- depth localization of lesions,
- post-stereotactic or ultrasound marker localization,
- alternative view to clarify possible lesion demonstrated on medio-lateral oblique,
- demonstration of the inframammary angle.

Area demonstrated

The majority of breast tissue with the exception of the axillary tail is viewed (**Figure 6.27, 6.28**).

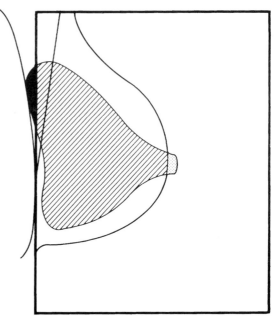

Figure 6.28 The area demonstrated.

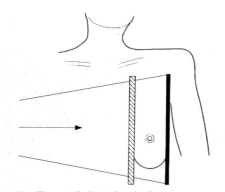

Figure 6.27 The medio-lateral projection.

Equipment position

The breast support table is vertical.

Anatomical position – left breast

The woman stands facing the machine with the lateral edge of the thorax in line with the film holder. Her left arm should be lifted and her hand placed on the handle bar. The breast should be in line with the centre of the support table (**Figure 6.29**).

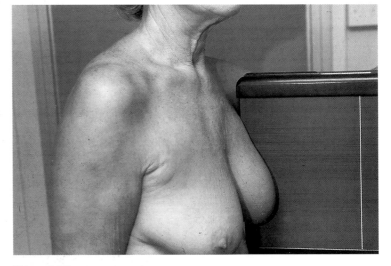

Figure 6.29

Breast positioning

1. Hold the upper humerus with your left hand. Using your right hand, lift the breast up and away from the chest wall. Leading with the nipple, encourage her to lean forward into the machine, allowing her elbow to bend as she moves forward (**Figure 6.30**).
   Check that:
   (a) the nipple is in profile,

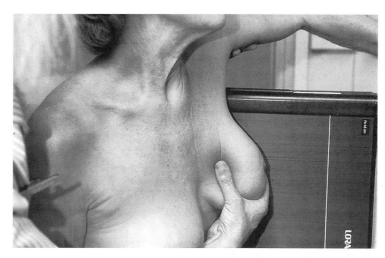

Figure 6.30

   (b) the inframammary angle is in view (**Figure 6.31**).

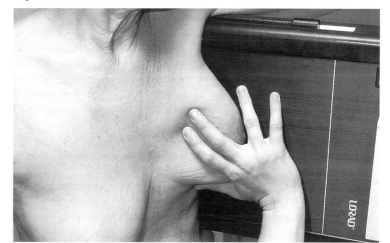

Figure 6.31

2. Using your right hand pull the upper portion of pectoral muscle forward onto the film, ensuring that the corner of the film is in the axilla (**Figure 6.32**).
3. Rest the woman's arm on top of the machine.
   Check that:
   (a) the nipple is still in profile,
   (b) the inframammary angle is still in view,

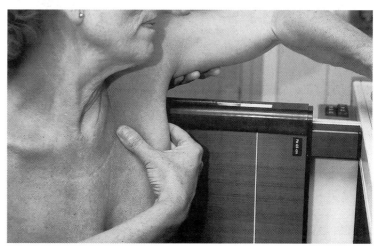

Figure 6.32

(c) the corner of the film holder is in the axilla (**Figure 6.33**).

Holding the left breast with your right hand and the left shoulder with your left hand, apply compression, expose and release.

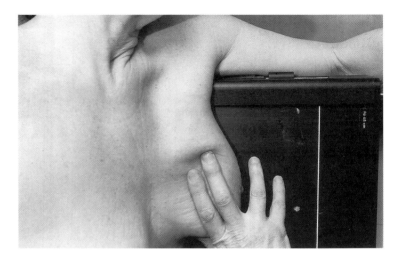

Figure 6.33

The latero-medial position and resultant mammogram are illustrated in **Figures 6.34** and **6.35**.

The medio-lateral projection should demonstrate:

* the nipple in profile,
* the inframammary angle,
* the lower part of the pectoral muscle.

Difficulties encountered

Applying compression in the latero-medial position is awkward for the radiographer due to the position of the tube housing.

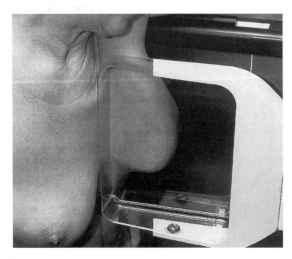

Figure 6.34 Breast in medio-lateral position.

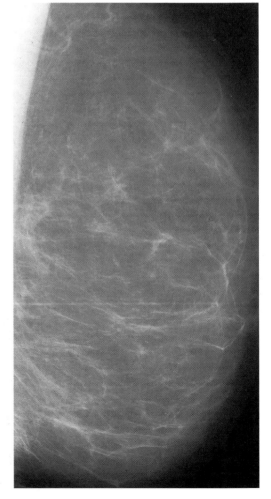

Figure 6.35 The medio-lateral mammogram.

LATERO-MEDIAL PROJECTION

Indications

This projection is used in the following circumstances:

- to demonstrate the medial quadrants,
- to demonstrate the inframammary angle,
- in the non-standard woman (see **Chapter 7**).

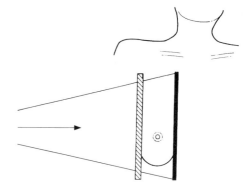

Area demonstrated

The majority of breast tissue, excluding the axillary tail, is shown (**Figures 6.36, 6.37**).

Figure 6.36 The latero-medial projection.

Equipment position

The breast support table is vertical.

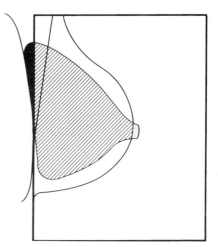

Figure 6.37 The area demonstrated.

Anatomical position – right breast

The woman is erect and faces the machine, about 2–3 cm back, with the table in line with her sternum. She should be asked to lift her right arm up and hold the bar on the tube column, keeping her elbow slightly bent (**Figure 6.38**).

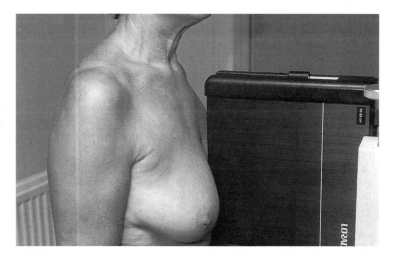

Figure 6.38

Breast positioning

1. Place your left hand on her right shoulder. Lift the right breast up and away from the chest wall with your right hand. Leading with the nipple, encourage her to lean towards the machine so that her sternum is against the support table (**Figure 6.39**).

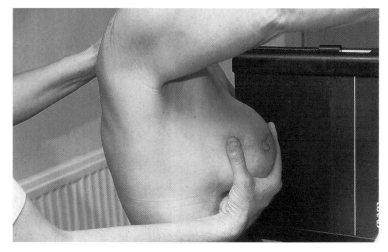

Figure 6.39

2. Encourage the woman to lean slightly to the medial and rest her forearm along the handle bar with the humerus parallel with the top of the film holder. Check that:
   (a) the inframammary angle is in view,
   (b) the nipple is in profile,
   (c) the anterior surface of the pectoral muscle is against the film holder.

Holding the right breast with the right hand and with your left hand on the upper dorsal region (**Figure 6.40**), apply compression, expose and release.

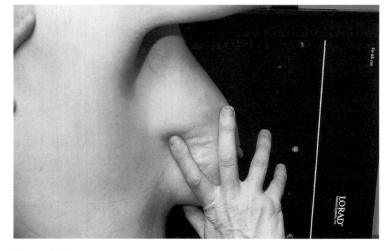

Figure 6.40

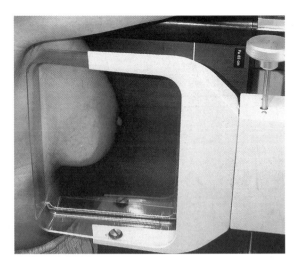

Figure 6.41   Breast in latero-medial position.

The latero-medial position and resultant mammogram are illustrated in **Figures 6.41** and **6.42**.

Difficulties encountered

Care must be taken that the compression plate does not get caught on the edge of the posterior axillary fold.

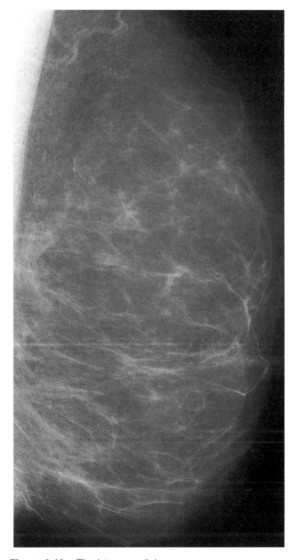

Figure 6.42   The latero-medial mammogram.

AXILLARY TAIL VIEW

Indications

This projection is useful for women with accessory breast tissue or the possibility of lymph gland involvement.

Area demonstrated

The high axillary region is viewed (**Figures 6.43, 6.44**).

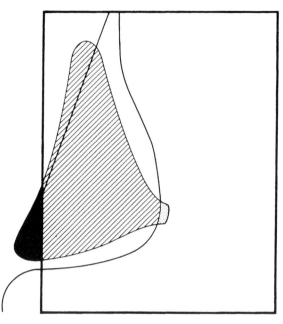

Figure 6.44　The area demonstrated.

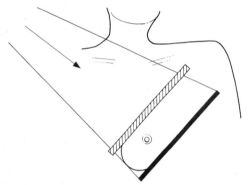

Figure 6.43　The axillary tail projection.

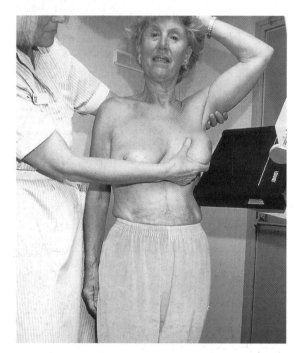

Figure 6.45

Anatomical position – left breast

The woman should face the machine with her feet at an angle of approximately 15 degrees. She should stand close to the machine with her hand on her head (**Figure 6.45**).

Equipment position

The table should be at 45 degrees from the horizontal and level with the notch beneath the end of the clavicle and the humeral head **when the arm is raised**.

Breast positioning

1. Lean the woman forward towards the machine, placing the corner of the table deep into the axilla (**Figure 6.46**). Do not be concerned with the lack of inframammary angle.

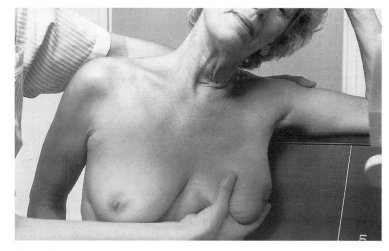

Figure 6.46

2. From behind the film holder, take hold of the woman's left arm and pull the arm and humeral head firmly across the top of the holder, ensuring that the corner of the film is deep in the axilla (**Figure 6.47**).

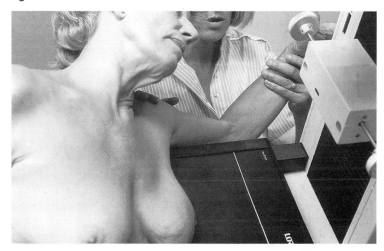

Figure 6.47

3. Rest her arm on top of the machine and encourage her to lean against the film holder. Hold the left breast forward with your right hand (this ensures even thickness of the breast to facilitate compression of the axillary region). Hold the left shoulder with the left hand (**Figure 6.48**). Encourage her to lean against the corner of the support table. Apply compression, expose and release.

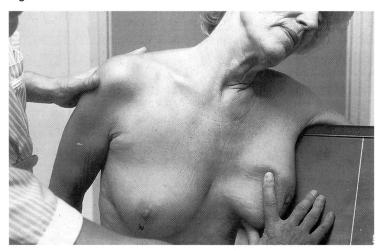

Figure 6.48

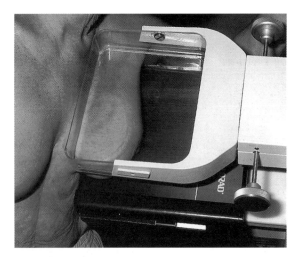

Figure 6.49   Breast in axillary tail position.

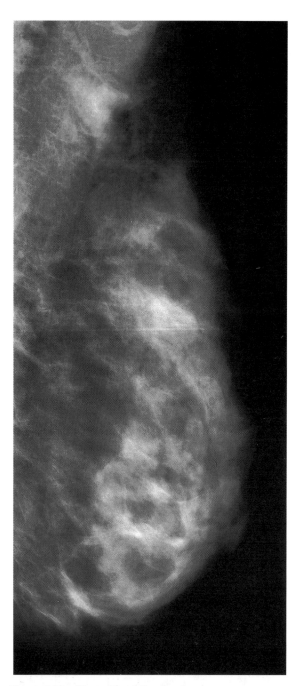

Figure 6.50   The axillary tail mammogram.

The axillary tail position and resultant mammogram are illustrated in **Figures 6.49** and **6.50**.

Difficulties encountered

Take care to avoid catching the humeral head or clavicle with the compression plate.

SPECIALIZED TECHNIQUES

These techniques are used when the basic projections have indicated a possible abnormality within the breast which requires further evaluation. Special projections are normally requested by the supervising radiologist, but it is helpful for radiographers to have a full understanding of their uses. In some departments the radiologist may delegate the responsibility for taking further views to the radiographer in his or her absence. This will save the woman from having two visits to the department and the increased anxiety this provokes.

Communication

A fully co-operative patient makes the task of achieving high-quality mammography much easier. For localized views, it is helpful to explain:

- what is being attempted,
- why it is being attempted,
- that the procedure is not easy, and that the woman's assistance and co-operation is essential if satisfactory images are to be obtained (i.e. it is a team effort).

Most women respond well to being shown the films and involved in the task, whatever the outcome (**Figure 6.51**). The radiographer should always take care, however, that she does not give an indication of the probable interpretation of the investigation, whether benign or malignant. The radiographer should not interpret the films for the woman nor offer false reassurance.

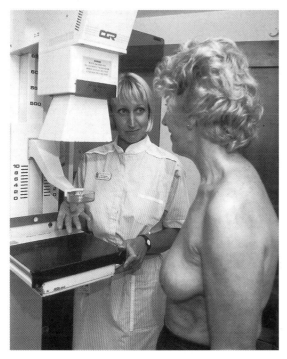

Figure 6.51

Positioning

Locating a small impalpable area in a large breast can be difficult. It must be recognized that time and care are required in order to minimize repeat films and associated stress levels for both patient and radiographer.

ROLLED VIEWS/DISPLACEMENT VIEWS

Rolled views can be performed in any projection. They are most commonly used in the cranio-caudal projection when superimposed tissue structures may be obscuring a lesion or may mimic a lesion. They can be a valuable alternative to paddle compression views which are explained in the section that follows. This technique can:

- project the superficial tissues away,
- expose the obscured areas,
- determine the reality of a lesion,
- demonstrate whether the lesion was superficial or deep.

A more acceptable technique might be to angle the tube 10 to 15 degrees which would reduce discomfort. A 'step oblique' method can also assist in demonstrating the reality of a lesion (Pearson et al 2000). When performing either rolled or displacement views the direction of roll, or tube swing, respectively, should be noted on the film.

LOCALIZED COMPRESSION OR 'PADDLE' VIEWS

Indications

Paddle views are used:

- to demonstrate whether a lesion is genuine or simply superimposition of normal tissue and/or
- to demonstrate whether a lesion has clearly defined or ill-defined borders.

Equipment required (Figure 6.52)

The following equipment is necessary:

- fine focus (highly desirable but not essential),
- moving grid,
- small compression paddle,
- AEC towards the chest wall,
- full field diaphragm (a full view of the breast will allow you to identify landmarks, make the necessary adjustments and improve visual perception).

The radiologist will generally select the paddle views required but, in his/her absence, the paddle views should be performed in the positions which demonstrate the possible lesion.

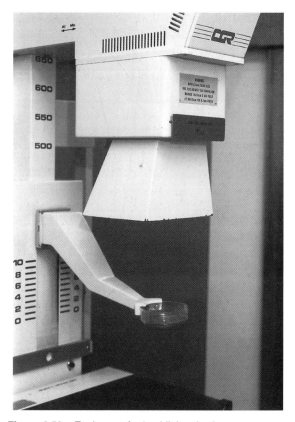

Figure 6.52   Equipment for 'paddle' projection.

Accurate localization of the area of interest (Figure 6.53)

The radiographer should:

- examine the original mammogram,
- measure and note down:
  - (a) the depth of the lesion from the nipple back towards the chest wall,
  - (b) the distance of the lesion above or below nipple level (or medial/lateral to),
  - (c) the distance from the skin surface to the lesion.

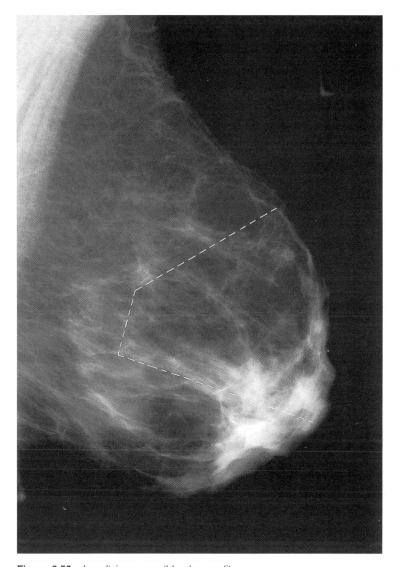

Figure 6.53 Localizing a possible abnormality.

Positioning (Figure 6.54)

1. Position the woman mimicking, as closely as possible, the positioning on the original mammogram.
2. Referring to the noted co-ordinates, move the woman until the appropriate portion of breast tissue lies over the automatic exposure device (AEC), and centred under the small paddle. **Remember:** make allowances for the fact that your measurements are taken from a fully compressed breast.
3. Begin to apply the compression.
4. Once the breast is held in position, but not fully compressed, check the co-ordinates.

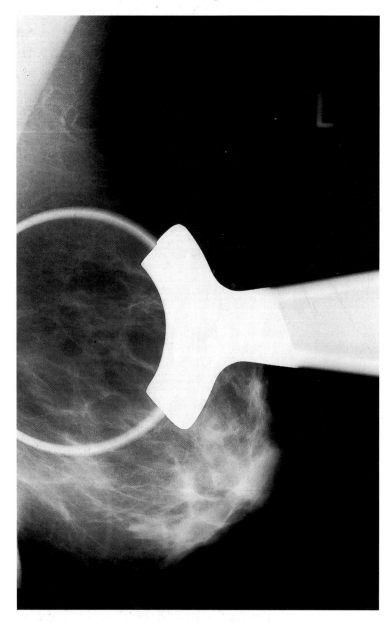

Figure 6.54 'Paddle' projection demonstrating that the 'abnormality' was simply superimposition shadowing.

5. If you are satisfied that the area of interest is beneath the paddle:
   (a) mark the centring point on the skin surface,
   (b) apply compression vigorously.
6. If not, adjust the woman's position until you are satisfied.

Compression force

With paddle views more vigorous compression than normal should be applied to the localized area (**Figure 6.55**). If the technique and the reason for the procedure have been explained to the patient sufficiently well she will tolerate this extra force without complaint.

Difficulties encountered

If the area of interest is not central to the small paddle it may be pushed out of the image field. A second attempt will be necessary.

MAGNIFICATION VIEWS
Indications

These are most often used to examine areas of calcification in order to establish their number and characteristics. Magnification views should be taken in the cranio-caudal and medio-lateral projections. The latter will demonstrate the 'teacup' effect typical of benign-type calcifications described in **Chapter 11**.

Equipment requirements (Figure 6.56)

The following equipment is required:

- fine focus (essential),
- magnification table,
- film holder (no bucky),
- small and large paddles,
- full field diaphragm.

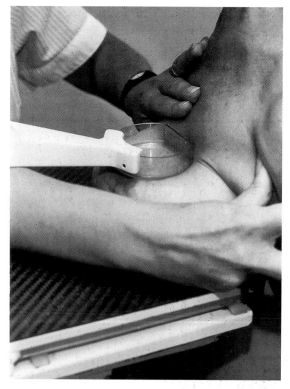

Figure 6.55

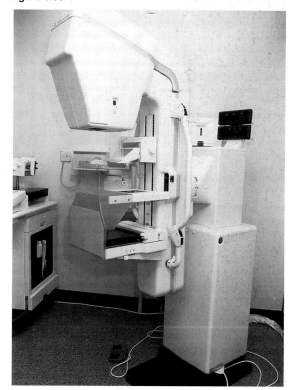

Figure 6.56   Equipment for magnification projections.

LOCALIZED/PADDLE MAGNIFICATION VIEWS

Small paddle magnification is generally most helpful in that compression can be applied more vigorously to the area of interest, improving contrast and definition. However, in cases where the calcification is extensive, a larger compression paddle can be used in order to visualize the whole area on one film. The measuring and positioning technique used for standard paddle views should again be utilized in order to locate the area of interest with accuracy.

FULL FIELD MAGNIFICATION VIEWS

The need to image the whole breast by magnification technique is relatively uncommon. It may be required in cases where there is likelihood of multifocal disease.

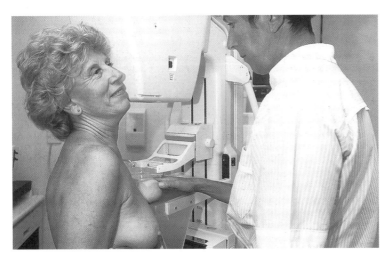

Figure 6.57

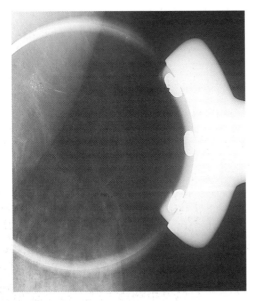

Figure 6.58 A lateral magnification view.

Exposure time

Due to the use of fine focus the exposure time will be considerably extended. It is advisable to ask the woman to stop breathing. (**N.B.** Do not ask the woman to breathe in and hold her breath! The expansion of the thorax will move the breast and your careful measuring will have been wasted!)

The final position is shown in **Figure 6.57** and the resultant mammogram in **Figure 6.58**.

STEREOTACTIC NEEDLE PROCEDURES AND MARKER LOCALIZATION

Stereotactic procedures can be performed within existing upright mammography equipment (**Figure 6.59**) with add-on features or specially purchased prone biopsy tables. Cost plays a major part in which system is available. Digital imaging is the method of choice for needle localization procedures (**Figure 6.60**). The use of digital imaging reduces the risk of movement and syncope as procedure time is reduced. Digital stereotaxis has also been demonstrated to increase diagnostic accuracy. Film screen systems with upright systems are still in use at the present time, in which case a fast processing cycle should be selected.

Whichever method and equipment is used the role of the mammographer cannot be over-

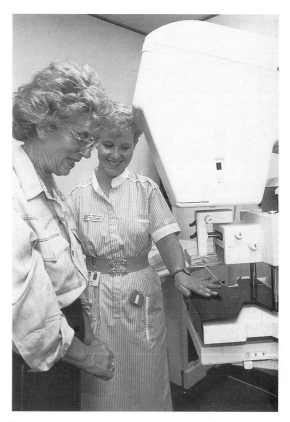

Figure 6.59 Explaining the procedure.

emphasized. Some key factors need to be observed in all stereotactic procedures:

- It is helpful if the mammographer has had contact with the patient before; rapport will have already been established and the mammographer will be familiar with the site of the lesion.
- Patient comfort is paramount if the procedure is to be successfully completed. The procedure must be undertaken with the patient seated comfortably in or suitably positioned on the prone table.
- If the patient is seated, this should be in a suitable chair with the lower lumbar area fully supported throughout the procedure so that the patient is not tempted to move.
- The lesion should be located as quickly and accurately as possible. This will minimize discomfort, unnecessary exposures and possible movement or syncope.

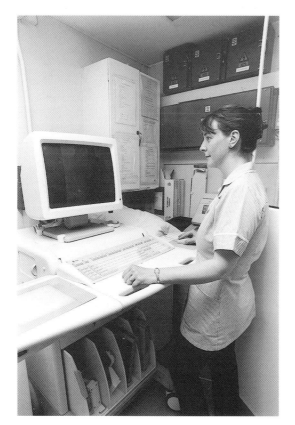

Figure 6.60 Digital stereotactic localization.

- Having positioned the woman, the outline of the 'window' in the compression plate can be drawn on the skin so that any subsequent movement of the breast will be evident.
- The patient should not be left alone while the procedure is underway.
- The mammographer should empathize with and support the woman throughout the procedure.

Core cut procedures

As core cut devices with firing mechanisms become more widely used for biopsy, the positioning skills of the mammographer have been increasingly challenged. Consideration should be given to the shortest route to the lesion and the distance between the lesion and the support table to allow for the throw of the needle by the device. Positions for this examination are more commonly one of the lateral or oblique projections.

Mammotome device

The Mammotome device is used with the needle parallel to the support table and the lesion is approached from the lateral. The positioning of the patient is more likely to be in the craniocaudal position.

SPECIMEN IMAGING
Core cut and Mammotome samples

In the last few years there has been a move away from the use of fine-needle aspiration cytology to increased use of 14 gauge core cut and 11 gauge Mammotome devices for diagnosis. As a result, the use of imaging for needle sample specimens has been introduced. Core biopsy and Mammotome specimen sampling need to take place within the department where the test is being performed. This will enable rapid identification of the presence of microcalcification and the need for possible further needle passes. Specimen radiography can be performed on a normal mammography machine, but the use of a specimen cabinet is a much better option although they can be very expensive.

Sample imaging on standard mammography equipment

- The specimen is placed on a small piece of card, in a sample container or in the lid of the specimen jar (**Figure 6.61**).

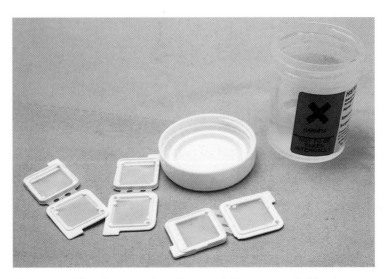

Figure 6.61 Specimen containers for 14 and 11 gauge needle biopsies.

- The specimen should be placed on the magnification table to introduce an air gap and enlarge the specimen to demonstrate any additional calcifications.
- The selected degree of magnification should be consistent for all specimens.

- Fine focus should be selected.
- Exposure factors will need to be set to the minimum. On some units the automatic exposure chambers can be used; on others, manual exposure parameters will need to be set. In either case, the kV should be set as low as possible.

Sample imaging with digital systems

This is a valuable and speedy practice and can give almost instant feedback on the success of the procedure (**Figure 6.62**). It is important to remember that a hard copy needs to be produced for inclusion in the patient's records unless the unit has a fully integrated image acquisition and storage system.

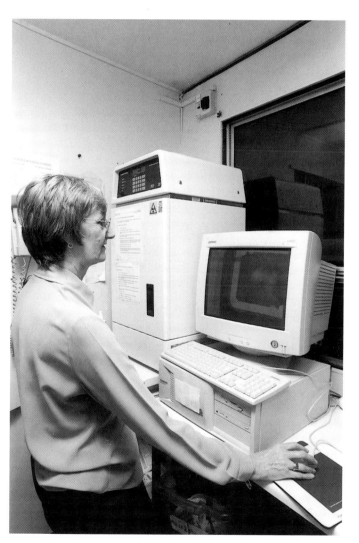

Figure 6.62   Viewing specimens with a digital specimen cabinet.

Imaging of excision biopsies

Excision biopsy imaging has been around for some time and was initially used in breast screening programmes when surgeons started excising small impalpable abnormalities and required confirmation of complete excision. This practice has now spread from screening services into symptomatic services since the benefits of establishing full excision with adequate margins has been demonstrated to reduce the number of second operative procedures and to reduce recurrence rates. Specimens are imaged within a compression device (**Figure 6.63**).

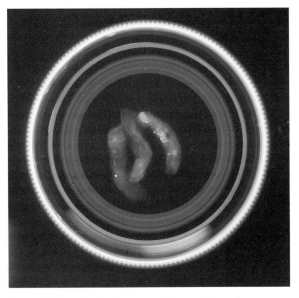

Figure 6.63   Needle biopsy specimen radiography.

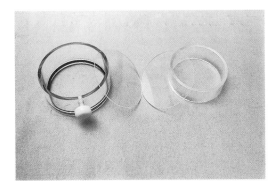

Figure 6.64   Diagnostic localization specimen containers.

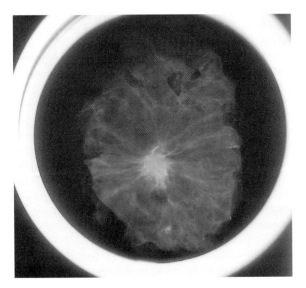

Figure 6.65   A diagnostic excision specimen radiograph.

Specimen cabinets in theatre are the best option and are extremely simple and safe to use (**Figure 6.64**). Image processing must be readily at hand so that the patient is not kept under anaesthetic longer than necessary. In this situation, the surgeon is able to make the decision as to the adequacy of the excision and further excise the margins if necessary before waking the patient.

Specimen radiography on a normal mammography machine is possible, but only advisable when no other alternative is available. The greater the distance that the machine and processor are from theatre, the longer the patient will remain under anaesthetic.

The advent of digital specimen cabinets is already influencing these procedures. In an ideal world the patient will be in surgery, the specimen imaged in theatre, the image sent to the radiologist's computer terminal who can confirm the presence or otherwise of the lesion. An intercom to theatre can inform the surgeon of whether further excision is required.

FURTHER READING AND REFERENCES

Andolina VF, Lille SL, Willison KM. *Mammography Imaging: a practical guide*. Philadelphia: JB Lippincott, 1992.

Logan WW, Janus J. Use of special mammographic views to maximize radiographic information. *Radiological Clinics of North America* 1987; **25**: 953–959.

Perason KL, Sickles EA, Frankel SD, Leung JW. Efficacy of step oblique mammography for confirmation of localisation of densities seen on one standard mammographic view. *American Journal of Radiology* 2000; **174** (3): 745–752.

Rickards MT. *Mammography Today for Radiographers*. Sydney: Central Sydney X-ray Programme, 1992.

Sickles EA. Practical solutions to common mammographic problems: tailoring the examination. *American Journal of Roentgenology* 1988; **151**: 31–39.

Wentz G. *Mammography for Radiologic Technologists*. New York: McGraw Hill, 1992.

7

Mammography – tailoring the examination

This chapter outlines how to optimize mammographic technique to suit:

- variations in breast development and shape,
- variations in chest wall shape,
- imaging of women with breast implants,
- imaging of the male breast.

THE INDIVIDUAL

As mentioned in previous chapters, most women experience some degree of embarrassment when undergoing mammography. For the woman who falls into the 'non-standard' category this embarrassment can be extreme. The radiographer must do everything in his/her power to reduce this embarrassment. The non-standard woman is a challenge to the mammographer and it is inevitable that it will take longer to examine her in order to obtain the best possible image. The more experienced the mammographer, the better he/she will be able to accomplish this.

This chapter provides some guidance on how to approach mammography in women with unusual chest and breast shape and size. There will be occasions when an individual does not fall into any particular category; it is then down to the mammographer's ingenuity to accomplish an adequate examination, bearing in mind the need to demonstrate all areas of the breast.

Should an adequate examination not be achieved after every effort has been made, the mammographer should advise the radiologist of the difficulties and that the whole breast may not have been imaged.

VARIATIONS IN BREAST DEVELOPMENT

Small breasts (Figure 7.1)

Small breasts can be difficult to image satisfactorily but some simple small changes in technique can be very effective in helping to achieve diagnostic images. The secret is in the selection of the correct angle and height of the mammography table.

Cranio-caudal projection

Raising the support table by 5–10 degrees at the lateral aspect may help to visualize the axillary tail.

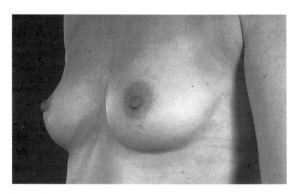

Figure 7.1

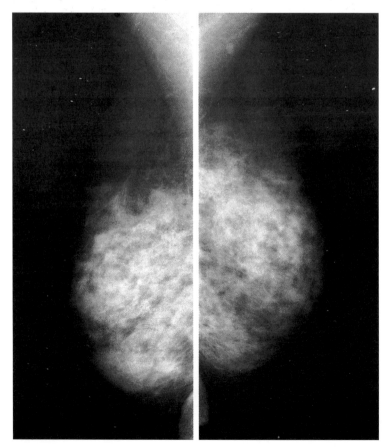

Figure 7.2

Medio-lateral oblique projection

The secret to performing a good quality medio-lateral oblique on the very small breast is the height of the machine. Any tension on the pectoral muscle (due to the film being high or anxiety on the woman's part) will make positioning very difficult. On rare occasions it may be necessary to use a manual exposure because the breast may not cover the AEC chamber on the small-breasted, small-stature woman. Consideration must also be given to the appropriate angle for each individual.

Figures 7.2 and **7.3** are mammograms of the same small-breasted woman. Comparing the two it is obvious that the image in **Figure 7.3** is significantly better; the improved image was achieved by correct selection of the machine height and angle.

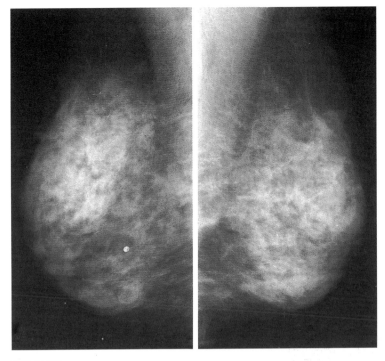

Figure 7.3

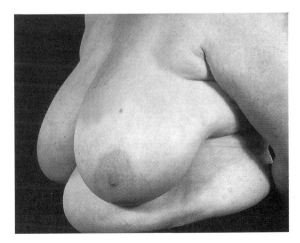

Figure 7.4

Large breasts (Figure 7.4)

Manipulating the large breast can be awkward for the mammographer. A large breast is difficult to lift and control with one hand and a mammographer with small hands may well have to use a two-handed technique to position the breast accurately. The technique for imaging the large breast will vary according to breast size and stature of the woman. The principle to remember is that all the breast should be imaged with some degree of overlap on each film. This overlap should be kept to 5–6 cm to minimize repeated irradiation to one or other portion of the breast.

Cranio-caudal projection

1. Stand the woman some 7–10 cm from the machine.
2. Ask the woman to stand up as straight and as tall as possible.
   These two manoeuvres help to lift the breast away from a protruding abdomen and make good positioning easier.
3. Lift the breast in the normal way onto the film holder.

If the breast is wide, imaging should consist of:

- a medially rotated cranio-caudal projection (see **Chapter 6**) (**Figure 7.5**),
- a laterally rotated cranio-caudal projection (**Figure 7.6**).

In each projection attempt to have the nipple in profile.

If the breast is long, imaging should include:

- a posterior cranio-caudal projection,
- an anterior cranio-caudal projection to include the nipple in profile (**Figure 7.7**).

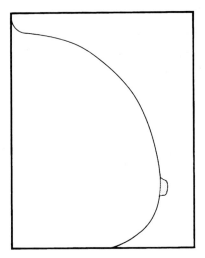

Figure 7.5 Medially rotated cranio-caudal projection.

When the breasts are very large, imaging should include:

- a laterally rotated cranio-caudal projection,
- a medially rotated cranio-caudal projection,
- a nipple view.

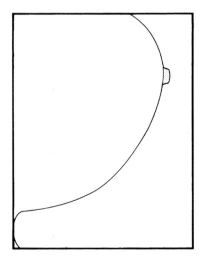

Figure 7.6 Laterally rotated cranio-caudal projection.

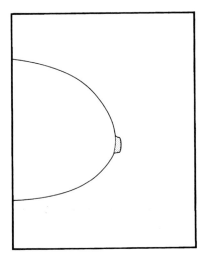

Figure 7.7 Anterior cranio-caudal projection.

Medio-lateral oblique projection

The technique is as follows:

1. Stand the woman 7–10 cm from the machine.
2. Ask her to stand as straight and tall as possible.
3. Adjust the height of the table in the usual manner (see **Chapter 5**).
4. Ask her to put her hand on her head.
5. Encouraging her to extend her lumbar region, and leading with the nipple, lean her into the machine.
6. Place the arm in the usual manner (see **Chapter 5**), taking particular care to eliminate excess skin and fat from the axillary region.
7. Lifting the breast up and away from the chest wall, examine the region of the inframammary angle.

If the breast is deep from clavicle to inframammary and the inframammary angle and lower border of the breast are excluded from the field, imaging should include:

- a superior oblique – see point 8 (**Figure 7.8**),
- an inferior oblique – see point 13 (**Figure 7.9**).

If the breast is long from the chest wall to the nipple and the inframammary angle and lower border are in the field, imaging should consist of:

- a posterior oblique – see point 20 (**Figure 7.10**),
- an anterior oblique – see point 23.

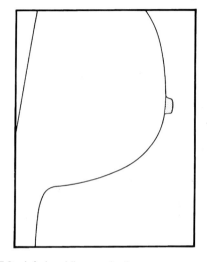

Figure 7.9   Inferior oblique projection.

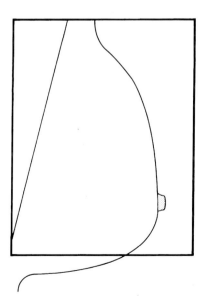

Figure 7.8   Superior oblique projection.

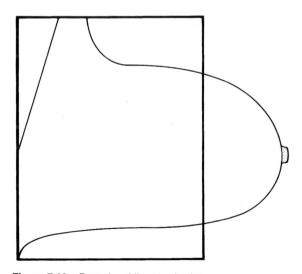

Figure 7.10   Posterior oblique projection.

When the breasts are very large imaging should consist of:

- a superior oblique,
- an inferior oblique,
- an anterior view to include the nipple in profile (**Figure 7.11**).

Superior oblique projection

Continuing from point 7 above, the technique is as follows:

8. Further extending her lumber region, withdraw the inframammary region and abdominal wall from the field.
9. Check for creases at the lateral border.
10. Lifting the breast up and away from the chest wall, spread the breast tissue across the film.
11. Check that the nipple is in profile.
12. Apply compression in the usual way, taking care that the breast tissue is compressed effectively.

If difficulties are encountered, adjust the position of the axilla to reduce the bulk of tissue.

Inferior oblique projection

DO NOT adjust the film height.

13. Stand the woman close to the film holder.
14. Leave her arm by her side.
15. Lift the breast up and away from the chest wall.
16. **Leading with the nipple**, lean the woman forward into the machine, keeping firm hold of the breast until the edge of the support table is at the mid axillary line. Check that:
    - the inframammary angle is clearly demonstrated,
    - the nipple is in profile,
    - there are no skin folds at the lateral aspect.
17. Lift the breast with the left hand up and away from the chest wall.
18. Remove excess tissue from the inframammary region, vigorously employing the technique described in **Chapter 5** (see **Figures 5.30–5.32**)

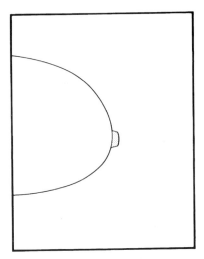

Figure 7.11 Anterior oblique projection.

19. Apply compression to the breast, maintaining control of the breast throughout.

In the **inferior** breast technique the compression force is used to enhance the 'lift' of the breast, thus helping to eliminate folds at the inframammary angle. The main body of the lower portion of the breast should lie a little **above** the centre of the film holder.

Posterior oblique projection

20. Using the technique described in **Chapter 5**, tidy the inframammary angle.
21. Lift the breast up and away from the chest wall.
22. Apply compression, ensuring that the compression applies to the breast and not only at the axilla.

Anterior oblique projection

23. Stand the woman 7–10 cm back from the machine.
24. Ask her to hold the handle bar so that she is steady.
25. Lift the distal part of the breast onto the film with the nipple in profile, allowing 1–2 cm overlap on the previous images.
26. Apply compression with care as the force will be applied to the most sensitive area of the breast.

Area demonstrated

The superior oblique projection should demonstrate:

- the pectoral muscle to nipple level,
- the pectoral muscle at correct angle,
- the nipple in profile.

The inframammary angle is **NOT** required on this view and this helps in excluding abdominal wall skin folds on the large woman.

The inferior oblique projection should demonstrate:

- the inframammary angle,
- the nipple in profile,
- the lower border of the pectoral muscle.

The posterior oblique projection should demonstrate:

- the full length of pectoral muscle,
- the pectoral muscle at the correct angle,
- the inframammary angle,
- the breast lifted with the ducts spread out and not drooping.

Anterior oblique projection should demonstrate:

- the nipple in profile,
- the anterior portion of the breast that is not visualized on the posterior view with some evident overlap.

Solid ball-shaped breast

The breast **must** be placed centrally on the compression plate to ensure that the compression maintains the breast in the correct position. In the oblique projection, in particular, if the centre of the compression plate makes contact above the centre of the breast disc, the compression will push one portion of the breast off the film. The inframammary angle is most commonly affected, as this is the point of least resistance.

Excessive compression on this type of breast, however well positioned, will ultimately push the breast out of the machine. The result is that insufficient length of pectoral muscle may be demonstrated.

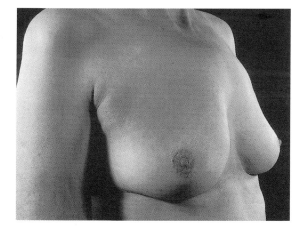

Figure 7.12

VARIATIONS IN THE CHEST WALL SKELETON

Prominent sternum (Figure 7.12)

Imaging in the oblique projection is not as difficult as is commonly believed. Frequently the breasts are more laterally pointing than usual and thus if the mammographer allows the woman to rotate her thorax medially a little, still leading with the nipple, an excellent result can be achieved.

In severe cases, two views may be necessary:

- a superior oblique, demonstrating the axilla, pectoral muscle, upper outer quadrant and the superior portion of the upper inner quadrant (**Figure 7.13**).

- an inferior oblique to demonstrate the infra-mammary angle, the lower inner and lower outer quadrants and the inferior portion of the upper medial quadrant (**Figure 7.14**).

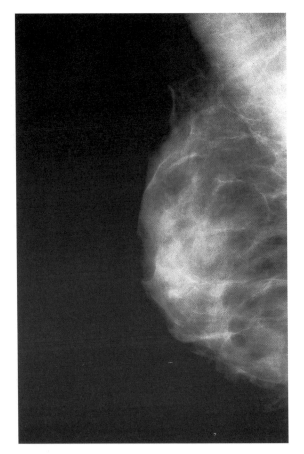

Figure 7.13

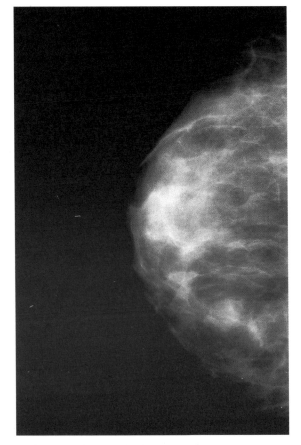

Figure 7.14

Depressed sternum (Figure 7.15)

Two views may again be necessary if the depression is great:

- a superior oblique,
- a latero-medial of the lower quadrants.

A latero-medial is chosen because the breast support table lies within the depression, facilitating visualization of the medial portion of the breast and the inframammary angle.

Prominent lower ribs

Cranio-caudal projection

It is difficult to achieve a good cranio-caudal in women with this skeletal variation. A slight elevation of the lateral side of the breast support table of some 10 degrees may be beneficial. The woman should be asked to lean forward as much as possible, from the waist, but not to the extent that her head gets in the radiation field. The nipple will frequently not be in profile.

Medio-lateral oblique

Flattening the film holder to between 35 and 40 degrees for the oblique will assist in positioning by allowing the film holder to be placed between the inframammary angle and the prominent portion of the ribs.

Unusual chest wall shape often means that it is not possible to position the AEC device in a satisfactory position to achieve the correct exposure. In these circumstances a manual exposure may enable the mammographer to accomplish the required coverage of the breast.

MAMMOGRAPHY IN WOMEN WITH BREAST IMPLANTS

Efficacy of mammography

The question of mammography on women with implants is a difficult one. Inevitably, as the implant is radio-opaque, visualization of all the breast tissue is often impossible. The policy adopted for imaging women with implants

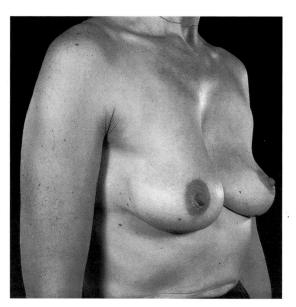

Figure 7.15

should be clearly defined by a locally or nationally agreed protocol. Women attending for mammography should be made aware that only limited examination may be possible and that, for them, breast self-examination plays an important part in the detection of breast abnormalities. Despite the limitations, many women with implants still wish to have mammography.

Anxieties in women with implants

The woman with implants is frequently embarrassed by the fact that she has implants, particularly if they were inserted for cosmetic reasons. She may be reluctant to admit that she has implants and, given an excellent cosmetic result, they may be difficult to recognize. She may also be anxious about rupturing the implants and considerable reassurance, that great care will be taken, will need to be given. Rupture of an implant as a result of performing mammography has not been reported. The mammographer should document in writing, with the patient's knowledge, the presence of any deformity or asymmetry of a prosthesis before performing mammography.

Having gained the woman's confidence, the mammographer should ascertain what proportion of the breast is formed by the prosthesis as this is important in deciding which technique should be used. The greater the proportion of the breast occupied by the implant the more difficult it is to obtain satisfactory mammograms. If more than 75% of the breast volume is occupied by the prosthesis, mammography is likely to be of limited diagnostic value and the radiologist may wish to perform breast ultrasound.

Positioning techniques

Each mammography service should have a predetermined policy for the examination of women with breast implants. The mammographer will need to evaluate the most appropriate technique to be employed for each individual:

- standard technique (**Figure 7.16 and 7.17**),
- Eklund technique (**Figure 7.18–7.20**),
- tangential views.

Standard techniques: Cranio-caudal projection (**Figure 7.16**)

Exposure factors A manual exposure will have to be selected and one cranio-caudal film taken initially to evaluate the exposure factors selected.

Breast positioning Breast positioning is as for routine cranio-caudal projection.

Compression Compression should only be applied to the level at which it will hold the breast in

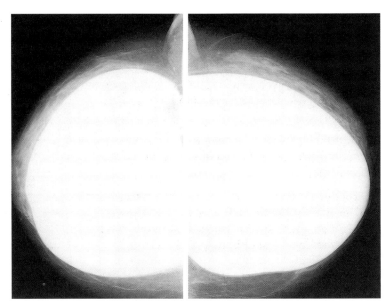

Figure 7.16

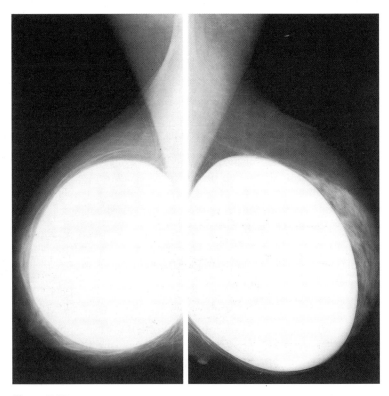

Figure 7.17

position. Further compression will not enhance film quality, and will simply cause discomfort to the woman and heighten any anxieties with regard to rupture of the implant.

The film is developed, the exposure factors evaluated and the examination repeated if necessary.

Standard techniques: Medio-lateral oblique (Figure 7.17)

Exposure factors   The exposure factor is increased by approximately one-third.

Breast positioning   Breast positioning is as for routine medio-lateral oblique projection.

Supplementary technique

If there is a large proportion of breast tissue to implant, the Eklund technique can be employed (Eklund et al 1988). This involves displacement of the implant to the back of the breast behind the compression plate with the result that only the breast tissue is compressed and imaged. This technique is particularly successful where the implant has been placed posterior to the pectoralis major. In these cases full demonstration of the breast tissue can be achieved.

The procedure is as follows.

1. Palpating the anterior border of the implant, pull the breast tissue forward onto the support table (**Figure 7.18**).

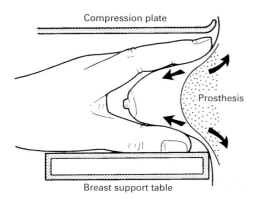

Figure 7.18

2. Ease the compression plate downwards onto the breast past the implant (**Figure 7.19**).

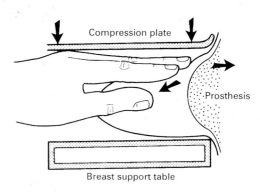

Figure 7.19

3. The anterior portion of the breast tissue is compressed and the implant pushed back towards the chest wall (**Figure 7.20**).

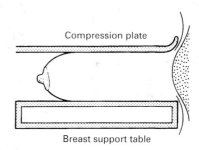

Figure 7.20

Tangential views

These should be performed in any woman with implants who is referred for mammography as part of the investigation of a localized lump in the breast.

MAMMOGRAPHY OF THE MALE BREAST (Figures 7.21 and 7.22)

Although not frequently requested, mammography of the male breast is occasionally required. The potential particular embarrassment of a man undergoing mammography must be recognized and the communication skills and professional manner of the mammographer in these particular circumstances cannot be overemphasized.

Practical difficulties encountered are:

- that the pectoral muscle is well developed and the breast tissue, as a general rule, is minimal. Accurate positioning, with the pectoral area not pulled excessively across the top of the film, will facilitate the application of compression,
- hair on the chest can also mean that the compression plate tends to slide down the skin surface but it will ultimately grip as it reaches the soft tissue of the breast itself.

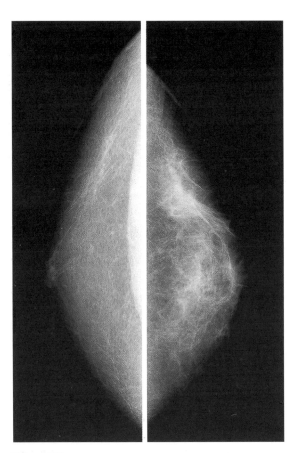

Figure 7.21

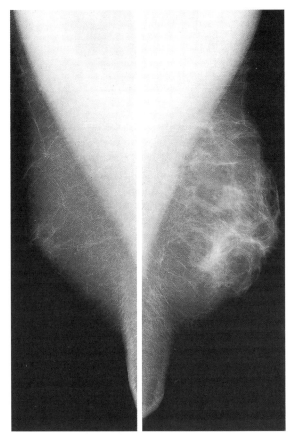

Figure 7.22

FURTHER READING

Breast Implants. Information for women considering breast implants. *www.doh.uk/bimplants*

Eklund GW, Busby RC, Miller SH, Job JS. Improved imaging of the augmented breast. *American Journal of Roentgenology* 1988; **151**: 469–473.

Kopans DB, Moore RH, McCarthy KA, Hall DA. Should women with implants or a history of treatment for breast cancer be excluded from screening mammography. *American Journal of Radiology* 1997; **168** (1): 29–31.

Logan WW, Janus J. Use of special mammographic views to maximise radiographic information. *Radiological Clinics of North America* 1987; **25**: 953–959.

Rickards MT. *Mammography Today for Radiographers*. Sydney: Central Sydney X-ray Programme, 1992.

Wentz G. *Mammography for Radiologic Technologists*. New York: McGraw Hill, 1992.

8

Radiological procedures

This chapter provides outlines of:
- why radiological procedures are carried out,
- the radiographic technical requirements of these procedures,
- the types of equipment used,
- the radiographer's role in these procedures,
- the complication of these procedures and what actions to take.

INTRODUCTION

The improvements in the technical quality of mammography and the widespread introduction of mammographic screening for asymptomatic women have both led to the detection of an increasing number of clinically impalpable breast abnormalities that require further radiological work-up to establish a diagnosis. The radiologist and radiographer have the joint responsibility of ensuring that all significant impalpable abnormalities are properly assessed. Initial assessment involves confirming that an abnormality is actually present using further mammography and breast ultrasound. The methods for doing so are discussed in **Chapter 11** and **Appendix 2**.

When the initial assessment process is complete the radiologist will have made a decision about the clinical importance of any abnormality found. This is usually done in the context of management protocols similar to those described in **Appendix 2**.

Impalpable abnormalities that show characteristically benign imaging features can be safely left without further intervention. However, many impalpable abnormalities have imaging features that cannot be called definitely benign and require some form of tissue diagnosis. Whenever possible this should be achieved without open surgical biopsy by using image-guided fine needle aspiration cytology (FNAC) and/or image-guided core biopsy. There are major advantages to women, and the clinicians managing their problem, in having a reliable cellular or tissue diagnosis at an early stage during assessment and this information will often obviate the need for open surgical biopsy.

There are two important reasons for obtaining a cytological or histological diagnosis by needle aspiration or core biopsy. Firstly, abnormalities that are very likely to be benign can be confirmed as such and surgical intervention can be avoided; women with these benign abnormalities can also be saved the anxiety of regular clinical and mammographic follow-up. A significant number of screen detected impalpable abnormalities fall into this category. Secondly, these techniques are invaluable in providing pre-operative confirmation of malignancy in abnormalities that have imaging features that demand open surgical biopsy. A pre-operative diagnosis means that women can be provided with fully informed

counselling and offered the most appropriate treatment choices; it also allows the surgeon to plan and perform surgery as a one-stage procedure, rather than diagnostic biopsy followed later by wider excision or mastectomy.

It is important that the radiographer has a full understanding of why and how localization of impalpable breast abnormalities are performed as they play an integral part in the process; radiologists rely on the expertise and skill of radiographers for the procedure to be successful.

Image-guided biopsy and pre-operative localization

Impalpable abnormalities can be localized for needle aspiration or core biopsy using x-ray-guided techniques or ultrasound. Ultrasound-guided biopsy is preferred as it is quick to perform, very accurate (with real time visualization of the abnormality while it is being sampled) and, most importantly, is associated with minimal patient discomfort and morbidity. The decision on which technique is used depends on the imaging characteristics of the abnormality being sampled. **Figure 8.1** shows the simple deci-

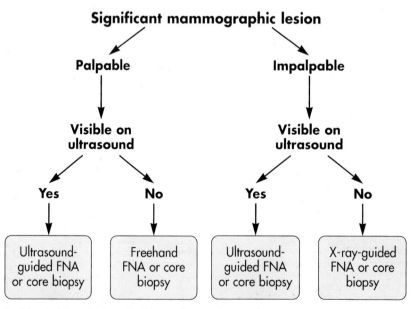

Figure 8.1 Flow chart for deciding which method to use for needle sampling.

Table 8.1 Imaging method for guiding localization of impalpable lesions according to type of mammographic abnormality

Mammographic abnormality	Ultrasound	X-ray guided
Masses	+++	+
Spiculate Abnormalities	+++	+
Deformities	++	+++
Calcifications	–	+++

sion making process and **Table 8.1** which technique is most suitable for the different types of mammographic abnormality.

If an abnormality is easily palpable, sampling is usually performed using ultrasound but, if this method fails to provide a diagnostic sample, repeat image-guided biopsy should be considered before going on to open biopsy. If an impalpable abnormality is clearly visible on ultrasound this is the guidance technique of first choice. However, x-ray-guided FNA should be used where there is any doubt about the ultrasound appearances – the radiologist must also be certain that the abnormality seen on ultrasound is the same as the abnormality seen on mammography or clinically palpable. If x-ray-guided core-biopsy is necessary there is no doubt that digital stereotactic equipment provides the greatest accuracy. The techniques used for image-guided sampling are very similar to those used to localize impalpable abnormalities for surgical excision.

X-RAY-GUIDED BIOPSY AND LOCALIZATION

The mammography room

The size and design of the room to be used for x-ray-guided procedures are important. The room chosen will need to be larger than a standard mammography room and should have sufficient space to accommodate with ease the mammography equipment and its accessories, the patient and up to three staff, but should not be so large that the patient feels vulnerable and exposed. Storage cupboards for biopsy and local-

ization items should be in the room so their contents are quickly and easily available. The room should be maintained at a temperature in which the patient will feel neither too hot nor too cold; optimal ambience is best achieved with an efficient air conditioning system. It is very important to ensure that the room temperature does not rise too high as this will increase the likelihood of the patient fainting during the procedure. Radiographers should be fully involved in the design and planning of any new mammography facility.

Preparing the patient

There are a number of tasks that should be completed before a patient undergoes a localization procedure. Image-guided procedures should be performed taking the shortest distance between the abnormality and the skin surface (**Figure 8.2**). This rule is particularly important for marker localization procedures for surgical excision performed using stereotactic equipment. In advance of the procedure a full set of mammograms including cranio-caudal and medio-lateral oblique are required for accurate assessment of which breast quadrant contains the abnormality:

- Abnormalities in the upper half of the breast should be localized in the cranio-caudal position.
- Abnormalities in the lower outer quadrant should be localized in the latero-medial position.

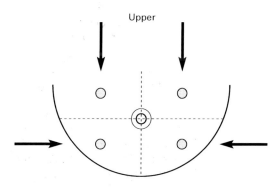

Figure 8.2 Approach for localization according to breast quadrant.

- Abnormalities in the lower inner quadrant of the breast should be localized in the medio-lateral or medio-lateral oblique position.

Not uncommonly none of these three basic positions are appropriate. An abnormality, such as parenchymal deformity, may be seen in only one projection; localization must then be performed using this projection. For this reason the procedure may need to be performed in the extended cranio-caudal position. In these circumstances detailed additional mammographic views should have been performed to allow the radiologist and radiographer together to decide on the most appropriate positioning. It is the radiographer, and not the radiologist, who has the difficult task of positioning the patient correctly for the procedure.

Similarly other medical conditions, such as cervical spondylosis or frozen shoulder, may preclude use of standard positions. In these circumstances the true lateral approach is often successful and is likely to be best tolerated.

Before any localization is undertaken the procedure must be explained simply and fully to the patient. The patient is much more likely to accept the procedure and co-operate if she has been informed of both why and how the test is performed. This may have been done beforehand by the clinician managing the patient but a repeat run through of the procedure immediately before it is performed is well advised and usually appreciated. Explanation is reassuring and helps to establish good rapport between the patient, the radiologist and the radiographer. The ambience should be relaxed with the patient aware and confident that the procedure is routine to the team carrying it out. The patient should be engaged in conversation as much as possible throughout with regular reminders of what is about to happen and frequent updates on how much longer the procedure is going to take.

The success of image-guided procedures is directly related to the skill and experience of the operators. The number of staff involved should be restricted, with a core of specially trained individuals undertaking all the procedures. Trainees must be closely supervised.

The number of staff involved in any one procedure should also be kept to a minimum. Ideally there should be three – the radiologist, the radiographer and a nurse (or another radiographer) to look after the patient. For certain procedures it may also be necessary for a pathologist or pathology technician to be present to prepare aspirates and other specimens. Patients do not appreciate too many staff being around unless they know who everyone is and why they are there. If trainees are involved the patient should be asked in advance if they mind them being present to observe – very few will object if asked politely. The patient must never be left unattended and should be supervised until the clinician has confirmed that the procedure has been completed and that the patient is fit to go. An examination couch with a head-down tilt facility should be available to lie the woman down on should she experience light-headedness or faint during or after the procedure (see complications below).

MAMMOGRAPHIC LOCALIZATION TECHNIQUES

There are a number of different techniques for performing x-ray-guided localization:

- Mammographic measurement,
- Modified compression plates
  - perforated plate,
  - co-ordinate grid,
- Purpose-made stereotactic devices
  - prone table,
  - erect breast support table.

Mammographic measurement

The simplest technique does not need any special equipment. The abnormality in the breast is localized by simple measurement of its position on cranio-caudal and lateral mammograms using the nipple as the reference point. Some radiographers and radiologists are masters of this simple technique but most agree that its accuracy is limited and unpredictable. With the current technology available this technique based on mammographic film measurement is not reliable

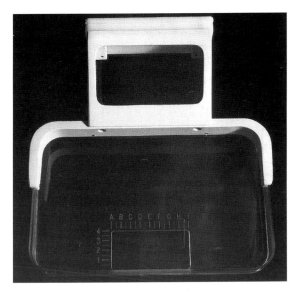

Figure 8.3 An example of a co-ordinate grid localization compression plate.

enough to be used as the basis for clinical treatment and cannot be recommended.

Modified compression plates

The simplest of these are modified perspex mammography compression paddles – the perforated plate and the co-ordinate grid plate (**Figure 8.3**). These paddles are attached to mammography units in the same way as conventional compression paddles with the abnormality localized by passing needles through the plate. Both the perforated plate and co-ordinate grid compression paddles are commercially available from most mammography unit manufacturers.

The quadrant of the breast containing the abnormality to be sampled or localized is identified from the lateral and cranio-caudal mammograms and the direction of approach chosen so that the shortest distance from the skin to the abnormality is taken, as previously described. The patient is then accompanied into the room and the procedure explained, including showing the patient the compression paddle and how the abnormality will be localized. The procedure is carried out with the patient seated in a specially designed chair (**Figure 8.4**) that is easily adjusted

for height and provides both lateral and back support. Chairs are also available that fold flat into a bed should the patient become lightheaded or faint during the procedure.

The breast is then compressed in the chosen position. If using the perforated plate a radio-opaque marker is placed in one of the holes close to the site of the abnormality as a reference marker. A film is then exposed and the relation of the abnormality to the perforations established. If the abnormality is not immediately under a perforation the patient can be repositioned and the process repeated. A needle (for biopsy or localization) is then placed into the breast through the perforation. The depth that the needle needs to be placed can be estimated from the original films. A film can be exposed with the needle in place to check its position – this is not always a reliable way of doing so because of inherent foreshortening.

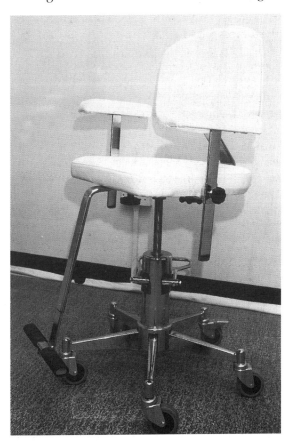

Figure 8.4 Chair suitable for localization procedures.

The technique for the co-ordinate grid is very similar. The breast is compressed and a film exposed to show the relation of the abnormality to the radio-opaque co-ordinates on the grid. The needle is then placed vertically down to the abnormality. Again the depth of the lesion within the breast can only be estimated and the position of the needle cannot be checked accurately.

Both the perforated plate and co-ordinate grid techniques are limited in their accuracy as the abnormality is localized in only two dimensions. These two techniques should only be used for localisation when dedicated stereotactic equipment is not available.

Stereotactic localization

Increasingly the results of sampling procedures are being used to decide patient management; women with benign abnormalities are told that excision is not required while women with malignant abnormalities are offered definitive treatment, including mastectomy, on the basis of the cytological or histological result alone. This means that image-guided fine needle aspiration and core biopsy must be extremely accurate and

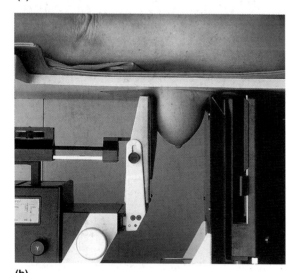

(a)

(b)

Figure 8.5 (a&b) Prone biopsy table.

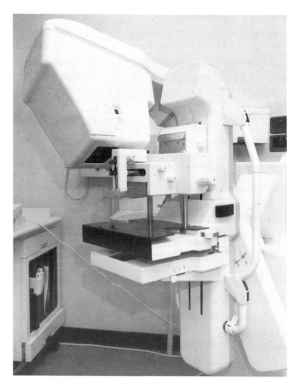

Figure 8.6 An upright stereotactic device attached to a conventional mammography unit.

the radiologist convinced that the correct area has been sampled. Stereotaxis is undoubtedly the most accurate of the currently available biopsy and localization techniques for impalpable breast abnormalities.

There are two types of stereotactic equipment. The first to be developed was a purpose-built biopsy table on which the patient lies prone (**Figure 8.5**). There are currently two commercially available tables of this type. The second type of stereotactic device is an accessory table which attaches to a conventional mammography unit (**Figure 8.6**). There are a number of different units of this type available and the majority use digital image acquisition.

THE PROCEDURE OF STEREOTACTIC LOCALIZATION

The radiographer should fully understand the technique of stereotactic localization. A brief step by step resumé is provided below. The procedure described is fine needle aspiration but the basic technique is the same for core biopsy and wire localization.

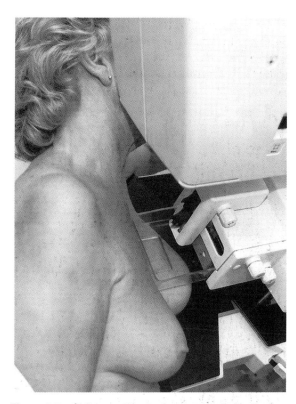

Figure 8.7   Oblique positioning for stereotactic localization.

The radiographer should:

- Check that the equipment and materials are correctly assembled before the woman arrives.
- Explain the method and purpose of the radiographic processes to the patient as they are performed. Using upright equipment the risk of the patient fainting during the procedure is considerably reduced if the patient is re-assured and relaxed.
- Position the patient and apply the compression plate after agreeing the ideal breast position with the radiologists (**Figure 8.7**). A marker pen should be used to draw the outline of the compression plate window on the skin (**Figure 8.8**). Movement of the breast under the compression plate during the procedure will then be easy to detect.
- Carry out the x-ray tube movements required to obtain the stereo images. For upright systems it is often necessary to place the patient's head in an awkward and uncomfortable posi-

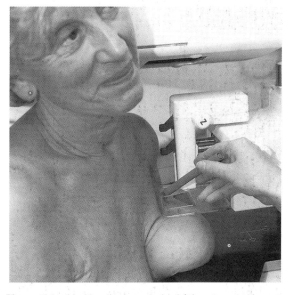

Figure 8.8   Marking the boundaries of the stereotactic compression plate window on the skin with a felt tip pen will allow you to easily see when the breast has moved under the plate.

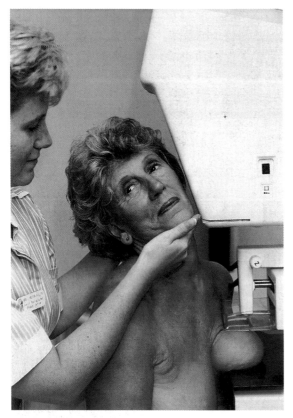

Figure 8.9 Careful positioning of the woman's head while the machine is rotated to obtain stereo images.

tion when the x-ray tube is being rotated. Care is required to avoid movement of the breast under the compression plate – the pen marks on the breast should be checked to ensure that their relationship to the compression plate window has not changed (**Figure 8.9**).

- The film should then be processed as quickly as possible. Check the stereo image with the radiologist. The patient should be repositioned if the abnormality is not clearly demonstrated or it is close to the margin of the compression plate window. It is better to reposition the patient than accept a sub-optimal position. For the depth calculation to be accurate **it is essential that exactly the same part of the abnormality is visible and selected on both the stereo images**. If the same point cannot be positioned under the left and right point markers because one lies more anteriorly then significant movement of the breast has occurred while the images were being obtained and further films will be required. The method of calculating co-ordinates using the stereo image varies considerably according to the make of equipment. This part of the procedure is therefore not described here.

Once a satisfactory stereo image has been obtained (**Figure 8.10**) and the co-ordinates of the abnormality calculated the radiologist will:

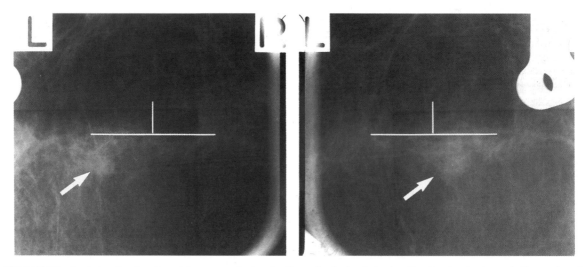

Figure 8.10 An example of a stereo image used for localization – the lesion to be localized is clearly shown in the centre of both images (arrows).

- Place the needle in the breast once the needle holder has been positioned correctly and after injection of local anaesthetic into the skin over the biopsy area. **Once the first needle has been placed a check film must be taken to confirm that the needle is in the correct position**.
- Check this film for correct positioning of the needle.

Aspiration may then be performed by applying suction and passing the needle up and down through the abnormality, rotating the needle during each pass to use the needle bevel as a cutting edge (**Figure 8.11**). Multiple passes may be made with each needle and the procedure repeated with several needles. The radiographer may be asked to assist by applying suction to the aspirating needle. If you are asked to do this remember that the **suction must be released before the needle is removed**.

Core biopsy is performed in a similar manner usually using a spring-loaded biopsy 'gun'

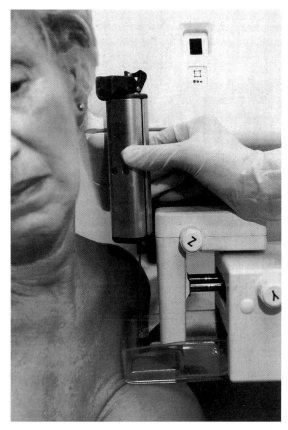

Figure 8.12 A spring-loaded core biopsy gun used for obtaining tissue samples for histological examination under stereotactic guidance.

(**Figure 8.12**) or vacuum-assisted mammography (**Figure 8.13**). The radiographic technique involved is the same as for aspiration and wire

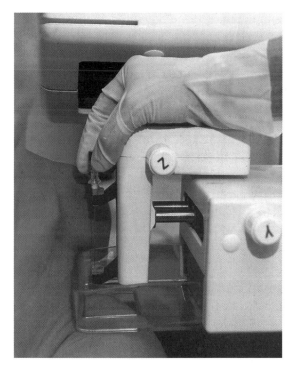

Figure 8.11 Fine needle aspiration being performed under stereotactic guidance.

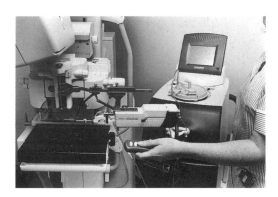

Figure 8.13 Upright digital stereotactic device set up for lateral approach vacuum-assisted mammotomy.

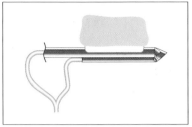

1 Stereotactic or ultrasound guidance used to position the probe

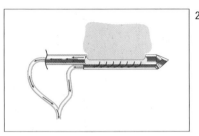

2 Tissue is gently vacuum aspirated into the aperture

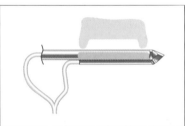

3 The rotating cutter is advanced, cutting and capturing a specimen

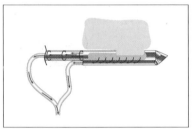

4 After the cutter has reached its full forward position, rotation and vacuum cease

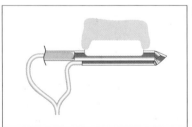

5 The cutter is withdrawn transporting the specimen to the tissue collection chamber while the outer probe remains in the breast

Figure 8.14 The principle of vacuum-assisted mammotomy.

localization. For vacuum-assisted mammotomy the lateral approach using a lateral arm probe holder offers some advantages for upright systems compared to the vertical approach (**Figure 8.13**). The lateral approach allows for accurate biopsy in smaller breasts where the compressed depth may be too small to allow for vertical biopsy and this technique also facilitates easier access to the retroareolar area and close to the chest wall. **Figure 8.14** shows the principle of vacuum-assisted mammotomy.

Stereotactic pre-operative marker localization

The procedure for marker localization is very similar to stereotactic fine needle aspiration and core biopsy. Stereotactic equipment is not essential for localization but does make the process more accurate. For diagnostic procedures localization must be as accurate as possible so that the surgeon can achieve the best possible cosmetic result. In the United Kingdom, National Health Service Breast Screening Programme surgical QA guidelines require that diagnostic biopsies

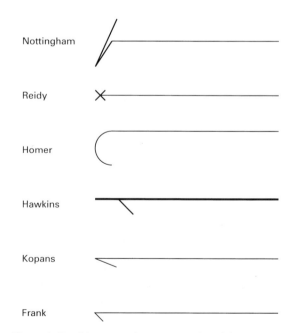

Figure 8.15 Diagrammatic representation of the more common marker wire types.

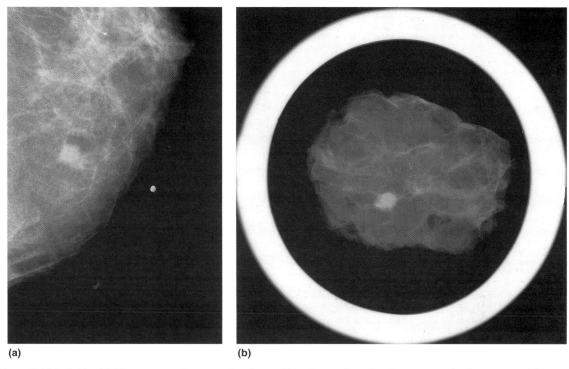

(a) (b)

Figure 8.16 (a & b)   (a) Mammogram demonstrating the position of a marker wire after stereotactic placement and (b) a specimen radiograph confirming wide excision after surgery.

should not weigh more than 20 g – about 2 cm in diameter. Surgeons appreciate accurate localization in these circumstances.

There are a large number of marker wires available (**Figure 8.15**). The choice of which wire to use ultimately rests with the surgeon performing the biopsy or excision. Lesions can also be marked with dye or carbon granules but these techniques are not favoured where accurate local excision is required. Many surgeons prefer localization techniques which allow them, rather than the radiologist, to choose the site for skin incision.

The single most important aspect of stereotactic localization is assessment of abnormality depth in the compressed breast. The aim should always be to place the marker through the abnormality. A surgeon will almost always be able to locate a lesion where the wire is placed too far through the lesion; the same is not true when the marker wire tip lies short of the lesion. It is essential to check the position of the wire in relation to

the abnormality in the breast after the marker procedure with mammography (**Figure 8.16**).

Helpful tips

- For all stereotactic procedures remember to mark the margins of the compression plate window on the breast with a marker pen (**Figure 8.8**). This makes it easy to spot when the breast has moved and that repositioning may be necessary. This often occurs when the stereo images are being obtained and the patient's head has to be turned awkwardly (**Figure 8.9**). Move the tube slowly and carefully while supporting the patient in position. If the breast does move in relation to the compression plate another set of stereo images will be required as the localization will not be accurate. Sometimes if the movement is excessive the breast will have to be repositioned under the compression plate.

• For core biopsy of an abnormality consisting of or containing calcifications the specimens can be x-rayed with magnification on a conventional mammography unit to confirm that a representative sample has been obtained. The exact techniques for doing this depend on the equipment used. As a rule manual exposure factors are used with the kV set at the lowest achievable to maximize tissue contrast. The specimen must be kept moist with saline to ensure that the tissue does not degrade and adversely affect subsequent histological examination.

Stereotactic procedures using a prone table

The prone biopsy table (**Figure 8.5**) was first developed at the Karolinska Institute in Sweden and has been used for many years. There is no doubt that this type of device is effective, particularly for biopsy procedures. The main difference compared to the other techniques already described is that the patient lies prone on a couch with the breast protruding through an aperture (**Figure 8.5**). There is no doubt that this position is more comfortable for the patient than the localization procedures already described. The woman is much more likely to tolerate the procedure, with light-headedness and syncope being much less commonly encountered. With discomfort of the woman much less of a factor the radiologist can apply the technique with less haste and may feel more able to perform repeated biopsies if necessary. Prone table devices are probably also easier to operate than other devices and there are some claims that they are more accurate.

Digital imaging is available for this type of equipment and will soon also be available for all mammography examinations. There is no doubt that a digital facility represents a major technological breakthrough. Digital processing significantly reduces the time required for stereotactic procedures. The major disadvantages of the prone biopsy table are its cost in comparison to stereotactic devices that attach to conventional mammography equipment and the space required for this dedicated equipment that is not in constant use.

Biopsy and localization materials

The exact requirements for each procedure will vary. A checklist of requirements for each technique should be posted in the examination room. A typical procedure trolley for biopsy or localization will have the following items laid out:

• plastic or latex gloves (for the protection of both the woman and operator),
• local anaesthetic agent,
• cleaning solution,
• basic procedures pack (2 galli pots, cotton wool buds and swabs – the contents will vary from hospital to hospital),
• 2 ml syringe and needles for injection of local anaesthetic,
• 25 gauge needle for injection of local anaesthetic,
• 10 or 20 ml syringe for aspiration,
• aspirating needles × 5 and/or
• core biopsy needles and biopsy gun and/or
• localization needle and wire,
• extension tube for aspiration,
• glass microscope slides and/or specimen transport medium,
• pencil for labelling slides.

Aseptic technique

The risk of introducing infection through carrying out image-guided procedures is minimal. However, these procedures should be carried out using aseptic technique. Gloves should be worn for the protection of the patient and staff. The equipment used must be thoroughly cleaned with bactericidal solution before and after each patient to ensure that the small risk of cross contamination with blood is eliminated. Advice on which solutions can be safely used on equipment is usually provided by the manufacturers, if not the hospital sterile supplies department or control of infection officer will give advice.

If you are involved in clearing up a trolley after a biopsy or localization procedure **make sure**

Table 8.2 Complications of image guided localization procedures

Complication	Patients affected
Severe Pain	0.5%
Severe Bleeding	0.1%
Light-headedness	3%
Syncope	1%

you are wearing plastic gloves and that you know how to dispose of sharps safely. Use forceps to pick up scalpel blades and do not disconnect needles from syringes–dispose of syringes in the sharp's receptacle with the needle still connected.

COMPLICATIONS

The complications that may occur during radiological mammographic procedures are listed in **Table 8.2**.

Complications are uncommon and are less likely to happen when the medical team performing the procedures is experienced in the techniques. It is the radiologist's and clinician's responsibility to ensure that the procedure to be performed is adequately explained to the patient and to ensure that there are no contraindications, such as anticoagulant therapy and allergy to local anaesthetic.

Pain and tenderness

Most of the pain associated with any needling procedure is caused by the puncturing of the skin, where the pain nerve endings are concentrated. This is usually limited to immediate sharp pain felt as the needle passes through the skin. Local anaesthetic can be used to anaesthetize the skin but the merits of its use must be decided for each procedure. If only a single fine-bore needle is going to be used then local anesthesia is probably not necessary, as the injection of the anaesthetic agent may be more painful than the needle biopsy itself. The pain associated with injection of local anaesthetic can be reduced by warming the anaesthetic fluid to body temperature before it is injected.

Bleeding and bruising

Slight bleeding occurs with virtually all needling procedures and is exacerbated by the hyperaemia and venous congestion caused by the compression of the breast used in the various x-ray techniques. About half of patients will develop a visible bruise at the site of needle puncture that will resolve over the next 5 to 7 days. Bruising is often accompanied by mild localized tenderness that subsides quickly and can be relieved by mild oral analgesia if necessary. To avoid unnecessary anxiety women should be warned that bruising and tenderness are likely to develop. A simple skin dressing, such as Elastoplast, should be applied to the puncture site (non-allergenic dressing for patients with allergy to adhesive plasters). This is simply to protect the patient's clothing from blood staining and the patient can be told to remove the dressing later the same day.

Bleeding may be more pronounced after core biopsy and pressure should be applied firmly to the puncture site for 3 to 5 minutes. The woman is often happy to apply the pressure herself. Bleeding can be minimized by using local anaesthetic combined with adrenaline. Significant bleeding is rare but can occur if a small blood vessel is inadvertently transfixed. Should significant bleeding occur during the procedure it should be suspended until the bleeding stops. Occasionally a procedure will need to be completely abandoned because of bleeding. Firm pressure should be applied to the puncture sight using the flat of the hand for at least 5 minutes or until bleeding stops. A pressure bandage can be applied but is rarely necessary.

Safety and blood spillage

As in any situation where some bleeding is inevitable all medical personnel likely to have direct contact should take all necessary precautions and wear protective plastic gloves. Care should be taken when cleaning and clearing away any items and areas where there has been blood spillage. All radiographers should be fully aware of and practice their unit's policy and guidelines on handling blood and blood-stained equipment. All equipment must be thoroughly cleaned and sterilized after each patient. Cleaning and sterilizing solutions should be compatible with the equipment – check the manufacturers' instructions. Every mammography assessment centre should have its own guidelines for these cleaning procedures.

Light-headedness and syncope

Light-headedness is relatively uncommon occurring in less than 3% of patients in our experience and is more likely when the room is humid and the temperature too high. Patients who complain of light-headedness during any procedure should be asked to breath slowly and deeply through the mouth. Most episodes can be relieved by this manoeuvre with progression to fainting avoided and the procedure completed successfully. Ask patients if they have experienced light-headedness or fainting during previous, similar procedures. If so, they are more likely to have similar problems again and it is wise to observe them closely. Engage them in conversation to distract attention throughout the procedure. Any patient who has experienced light-headedness should be asked to lie down for a short while afterwards until the supervising radiologist or clinician is happy that they have fully recovered.

In a small number of women light-headedness will progress to fainting (syncope). Women complaining of light-headedness must be closely observed and the procedure abandoned at the first sign of fainting. In these circumstances the patient should be laid down in the recovery position with her head placed lower than the body and legs. Most patients recover consciousness very quickly and should be offered ample reassurance as they do so. They should be encouraged to remain lying for at least 15 minutes. Again patients should only be allowed to leave after being checked over by the supervising radiologist or clinician.

REFERENCES AND FURTHER READING

Flowers C. (Ed.) *Image guided core biopsy of the breast: a practical approach*. Greenwich Medical Media, London, 1998.

Heywang-Kobrunner SH, Scheer I, Dershaw DD. *Diagnostic Breast Imaging*. Thieme, New York, 1997.

Kopans DB. *Breast Imaging* (second edition). Lippincott-Raven, Philadelphia, 1998.

Litherland J. The role of needle biopsy in the diagnosis of breast lesions. *The Breast* 2001; **10**: 383–387.

Michell MJ. Image guided breast biopsy: technical advances. *British Journal of Radiology* 1998; **71**: 908–909.

Parker SH, Stavros AT, Dennis MA. Needle biopsy techniques. *Radiological Clinics of North America* 1995; **33**: 1171–1186.

Teh W, Evans AJ, Wilson ARM. Editorial. Definitive non-surgical breast diagnosis: the role of the radiologist. *Clinical Radiology* 1998; **53**: 81–84.

9

Training, education and continuing professional development in mammographic practice

This chapter outlines:

- training and education requirements for radiographers,
- specialist education for radiographers in mammography,
- role development opportunities,
- auditing clinical practice.

TRAINING AND EDUCATION FOR RADIOGRAPHERS IN MAMMOGRAPHY

For the last 12 to 13 years the Society and College of Radiographers, the UK professional body, has awarded a Certificate of Competence in Mammography to state-registered radiographers who have achieved the required standards for mammography. The Certificate of Competence in Mammography is held in high regard by UK radiographers and those from abroad. Until recently the qualification was set at post diplomat level. This reflected the fact that the majority of state-registered radiographers had been qualified in previous years with the College of Radiographers Diploma of Radiography. Since 1990 radiography education has gradually been taken forward into a graduate framework (**Figure 9.1**). In the last 5 years all radiographers have qualified at degree level. This change has moved the radiography profession forward developing skills of research, evaluation, reflection and evidence-based practice.

To reflect the needs of graduate radiographers, training and education relating to additional

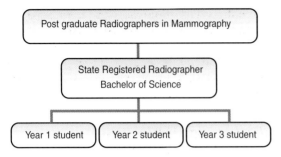

Figure 9.1 Training and education route for radiographers in mammography.

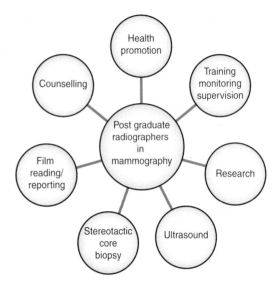

Figure 9.2 An example of a few of the professional development opportunities in mammography.

specialist skills need to be placed in a postgraduate framework. The first postgraduate mammography course was validated by the Society of Radiographers in 1995; since then all other mammography training and education institutions have followed this lead. The Society of Radiographers recently published new guidelines for universities and clinical departments on the requirements for postgraduate mammography courses.

Moving from post-diplomat to post-graduate or Masters degree training and education has required radiographers to have not only in-depth knowledge of mammography and mammographic services, but also the ability to research best practice in both mammography and the wider diagnostic service. State-registered radiographers in mammography are now equipped not only to provide a high-quality clinical mammography service but also to be enquiring and proactive practitioners who can influence the service from an evidence base.

EXPANDING THE ROLE OF THE POST GRADUATE MAMMOGRAPHER

Subsequent to these developments, courses have been developed in areas of advanced clinical practice. These are generally modular in format and offer students courses that will reflect their personal needs and those of their service. Radiographers are now moving to obtaining Masters degrees in either advanced clinical practice or management. Courses offer a variety of modules such as film reading/interpretation, ultrasound and needle biopsy and are validated

and accredited by the Society of Radiographers and the academic institution (**Figure 9.2**).

Radiographers who have successfully completed courses in advanced clinical skills have gained the respect of their medical colleagues for their demonstrable additional skills and are now practicing alongside them. These developments will enable radiographers to take a more proactive role in service delivery. Many radiographers both in the UK and further field are taking on advanced roles in film reading interpretation, ultrasound, needle biopsy, counselling, health promotion and many other areas.

WORKFORCE PRESSURES

At the present time there is evidence of growing shortages of both qualified radiographers and radiologists. In the past few years there has been an increasing demand for mammography services and this demand is expected to continue as a result of the demographic increases, heightened breast awareness amongst the population and the expansion and extension of the UK breast screening programme. The increased workload and ever-reducing staff numbers will create tremendous pressures on the diagnostic service. Unless an additional workforce is identified to address the increased service, breast diagnosis will be delayed. This will also create barriers to role development at a time when the opportunity has finally arrived to move beyond the traditional boundaries of radiography.

The recent revisions to the Ionising Radiation Regulations, IR(ME)R 2000 provide opportunities for state-registered radiographers to take greater responsibility and accountability within the service. These regulations also allow the use of non-state-registered practitioners working under the supervision of a state-registered practitioner. The non-state-registered practitioners will have to be suitably trained and deemed competent. This review of the rules governing irradiating patients has led to the development of a potential additional radiographic workforce.

A proposal has been put forward to employ support staff to undertake training in specific radiographic practices under the supervision of a state-registered radiographer (**Figure 9.3**). The first service in which this is being piloted is the mammography service. Whilst the pilot is taking place, competency statements are being devised against which clinical performance can be audited. This will ensure that the introduction of the assistant grade does not in any way compromise patient care. Once this pilot has been fully evaluated there is a potential for this to be used in other mammography services and within the wider diagnostic field where recruitment of state-registered radiographers and/or consultant radiologists is proving difficult. Recruitment of sufficient staff to perform the mammographic

examinations will allow radiographers to expand and extend their role in areas of personal interest and aptitude. The intention is that support staff will eventually enter a radiography degree course leading ultimately to an increase in state-registered radiographers.

AUDITING MAMMOGRAPHIC CLINICAL PRACTICE

For an autonomous profession auditing clinical practice is essential. Each mammography practitioner needs to review and reflect on clinical practice as part of regular personal performance monitoring. Continued monitoring of mammographic skills will help to maintain and improve the quality of service provided to clients. Attaining and maintaining high-level clinical skills will not occur without the continued pursuit of excellence. Bearing in mind the possible introduction of an assistant grade, the continued audit of mammographic performance for all practitioners is imperative. To facilitate audit of personal performance, mammography practitioners should clearly identify their own work by placing a marker on each film. This can either be their initials or a number specific to them. It should be placed at the lateral/axillary aspect and distant from the woman together with the orientation markers.

Review of repeated examinations

One method is to review repeat and recall rates. The standard set for the mammographers is that the proportion of repeat examinations should not exceed 3%. This is important so that radiation dose is kept to a minimum and that repeat films do not raise patients anxiety and potentially deter women from subsequent attendance for breast screening.

Repeat films can provide evidence of both equipment issues and mammographer performance. Regular monitoring will provide opportunities for remedial action in both areas. If the technical recall rate is due to equipment malfunction the frequency of this should be noted and the equipment taken out of service if films are likely to be undiagnostic.

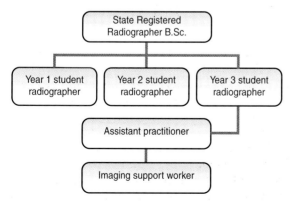

Figure 9.3   Alternative route into radiography.

In the case of repeat films due to the technical skills of the mammographer performing the examination, reviewing the work will identify trends in practice and identify any further training needs.

The P, G, M and I system

In 1993 performance criteria and a grading system for mammographic practice were introduced and incorporated into the training syllabus and the quality assurance guidelines for mammography. This was commonly called the 'P, G, M and I system' (**Table 9.1**). The implementation of this system was met with some apprehension but over time it was implemented throughout the UK both for training and ongoing performance monitoring. This system has also been widely adopted since then by Australia, New Zealand and Hong Kong. The great strengths and benefits of this system were that a clear standard for mammography clinical prac-

Table 9.1   P, G, M and I system

Criteria for image assessment of medio-lateral oblique	Criteria for image assessment of cranio-caudal projection oblique classification of images
1. Whole breast imaged Pectoral muscle shadow to nipple level Pectoral muscle at correct angle Nipple in profile Inframammary angle clearly demonstrated **2.** Correct annotations clearly shown Woman's identification Anatomical markers Positional markers (if used) Radiographer identified Date of examination **3.** Correct exposure according to working practice **4.** Adequate compression **5.** Absence of movement **6.** Correct processing **7.** Absence of processing and handling artefacts **8.** Skin fold free **9.** Symmetrical images	**P = Perfect Images** Both images meet all the listed criteria and will be categorized as **P** images. **G = Good Images** Both images meet all the listed criteria inclusive of numbers 1–6 and will be categorized as **G** images. 7, 8 and 9 in *minor degree* will be categorized as **G** images. **M = Moderate Images** Acceptable for diagnostic purposes: **1.** Pectoral muscle not to nipple level but back of breast adequately shown **2.** Pectoral muscle not at correct angle but back of breast adequately shown **3.** Nipple not in profile but retroareolar region well demonstrated **4.** Inframammary angle not clearly demonstrated but breast adequately shown **5.** Correct annotation **6.** Correct exposure according to working practice **7.** Adequate compression **8.** Absence of movement **9.** Processing and handling artefacts providing the image is not obscured **10.** Severe skin folds providing the image is not obscured **I = Inadequate Images** **1.** Part of the breast not imaged **2.** Inadequate compression, resulting underexposed and/or blurred image **3.** Incorrect exposure – giving undiagnostic images **4.** Incorrect processing – leading to undiagnostic images **5.** Overlying artefacts including skin folds obscuring the image **6.** Inadequate identification **Quality Standards for Mammography** 97% of images to be in **P**; **G** or **M** category with not less than 75% in **P** and **G** Group <3% of images to be in **I** Group

tice was established and that the constant striving to achieve films in the 'Perfect' and 'Good' categories had a marked effect in raising the quality of mammography. Another strength of the system was that radiographers reviewed a whole series of examinations from both their own clinical practice and that of their mammography colleagues on a regular basis. This enabled informal comparisons to be made, discussions to take place and practice to be influenced.

In recent years the value and use of the P, G, M and I system has been questioned. Research has indicated that the scoring was subjective and that different individual practitioners produced different scores on the same sets of films. This can make inter-individual, unit or regional comparisons difficult. A further criticism of the P, G, M and I system is that it only covers the medio-lateral oblique projection. As all basic mammographic examinations include both cranio-caudal and medio-lateral oblique projections the criteria for high-quality work in the cranio-caudal projection should also be examined. Professional judgement will be needed to evaluate the whole examination. If an area is not evident on one projection it may be clearly demonstrated on the other projection. The ideal is to have a high-quality examination in which each pair of cranio-caudal or oblique images is matching in positioning and criteria and that the whole examination is of high quality.

Despite these criticisms, the system is not without its merits nor its supporters. Until such time as a suitable alternative is found or a system that can encompass two views is developed the P, G, M amd I system, or derivatives of it, will continue to be used in the majority of mammography departments both in training and on-going performance monitoring.

Reviewing mammograms

Examining a mammographic examination and comparing left and right projections can help in identifying positioning errors. This technique relies heavily on the understanding of the mammographer relating what is happening to the breast and the body whilst positioning takes place and how compression affects the breast tissue. This skill takes some time to develop, but once gained turns a competent mammographer into an expert one. Common quality factors for discussion in all examinations are:

- absence of movement,
- adequate compression,
- correct annotations,
- correct exposure,
- correct processing,
- absence of artefacts,
- symmetrical images,
- nipples in profile,
- skin fold free,
- whole breast imaged.

Others topics of discussion relate to the specific projection. For example, discussions about technique factors in the cranio-caudal projection could be:

- evidence of pectoral muscle at the back of the film,
- position of the pectoral muscle if evident,
- relationship between the posterior nipple line and the back of the film,
- demonstration of medial and lateral borders,
- depth of the examination from nipple to back of the film.

For the medio-lateral oblique projection discussions would include:

- height of the machine,
- relationship between the length of the pectoral muscle and the level of the nipple,
- the angle of the pectoral muscle,
- demonstration and openness of inframammary angle.

A series of mammographic examinations, image grading and discussion points relating to positioning factors can be found below (**Figures 9.4–9.16**).

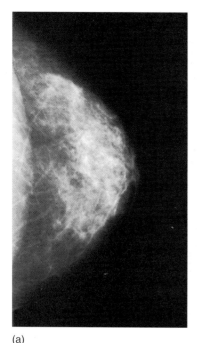

(a)

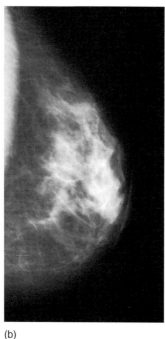

(b)

Figure 9.4 (a) and (b) (a) A very well positioned cranio-caudal projection. The nipple is central to the film and the posterior nipple line is at 90 degrees to the back of the film. The shoulder is relaxed hence the slightly elongated lateral aspect of the breast. The pectoral muscle is displayed at the centre of the breast disc directly behind the nipple. This confirms that the breast is correctly orientated. (b) The lateral border is excessively lengthy and the muscle tends to be in the lateral portion of the breast. This indicates that the woman has been rotated to the medial and therefore some of the medial portion of the breast will have been excluded.

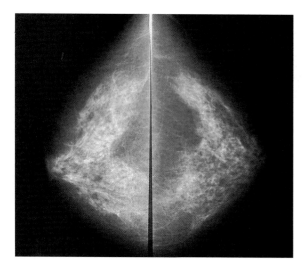

Figure 9.5 The left side is better positioned than the right. On the right there is some indication of rotation which has resulted in the shoulder obscuring the far lateral and exclusion of the ducts at the medial aspect

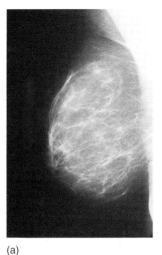

(a)

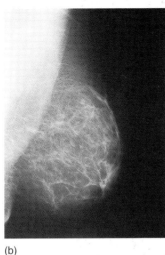

(b)

Figure 9.6 (a) and (b) Both these images are of the same woman. The films are under-penetrated by current standards. These films are included to demonstrate specific features.

(a) This shows a concave muscle. This could be due to physical tension but the effect is rather extreme and would indicate that the mammographer did not check to see that the skin at the lateral edge was pulled through completely prior to compression. The upper outer quadrant may not have been fully included.

(b) This shows a convex muscle. It has been suggested that this indicates a relaxed muscle. This is incorrect. The muscle takes on this appearance when positioning is not optimal and there is considerable bulk in the upper outer quadrant region. When compression is applied the plate has to press against this bulk rather than the breast and the pressure pulls and drags the muscle forward. The risks are that the woman experiences extreme discomfort in the upper region and that compression is not effective in the lower portion of the breast. The ducts will then have a drooping appearance and may be blurred.

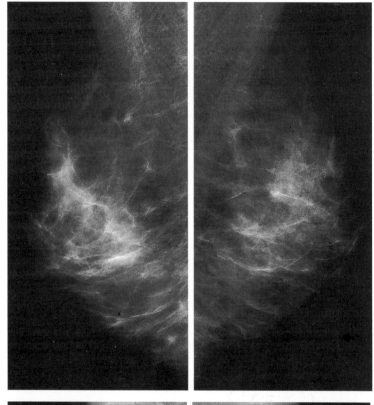

Figure 9.7 Perfect obliques.

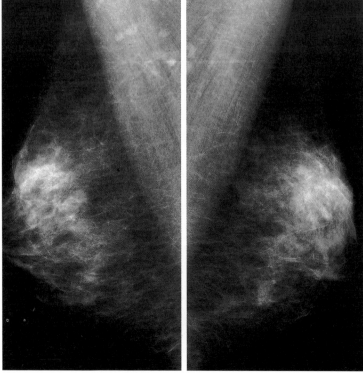

Figure 9.8 Perfect obliques.

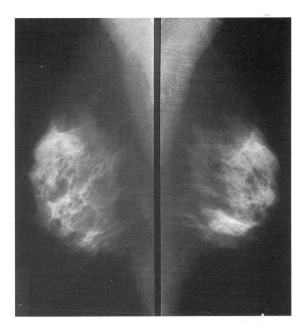

Figure 9.9 Good obliques. Slight crease on right side at the back of the film.

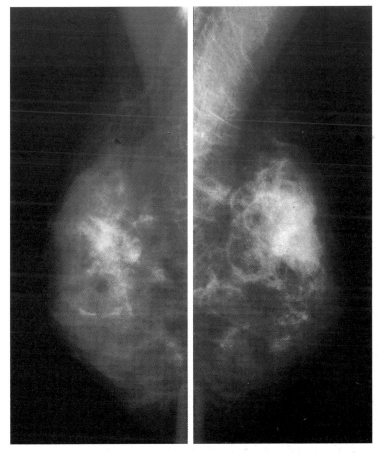

Figure 9.10 Good obliques. Both are fairly good examinations. It is the differences as well as the common good points that merit discussion. The muscle on the right is not quite over far enough. The one on the left is over a little too much. The ideal is probably somewhere in between. The film is under-penetrated on the left. This may be due to the difference in the involutionary pattern and has resulted in the AEC being beneath dense breast tissue on the right but not on the left. The difference in positioning may also have been a factor, as compression will not have been applied so easily on the left. Both inframammary angles are on but are creased. This area is behind the area visible to the mammographer. The technique outlined in **Figures 5.29 to 5.33** needs to be utilized.

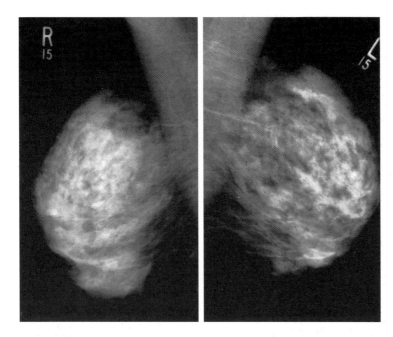

Figure 9.11 Good obliques. The left side is very well positioned for a woman of this build. The right side is not quite as good. The arm has been pulled over further or the woman has been allowed to place her hand in a slightly different position to that taken for the left oblique. As a result the right breast is not as well lifted as on the left. It is also noteworthy that close examination of the muscle on the right side demonstrates the pectoralis major and minor.

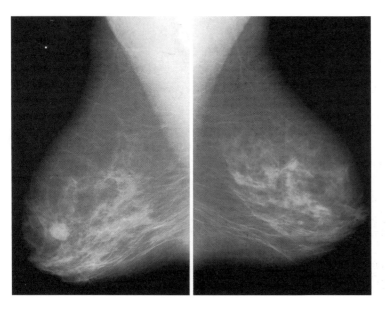

Figure 9.12 Moderate obliques. The left oblique is in a reasonable position. All the essential criteria are present indicating the whole breast has been imaged. The breast tissue itself is well demonstrated as the ducts are all leading towards the nipple in lines similar to the segments of an orange. There is no indication of breast droop. The muscle is a little tense. The right side however, is different, the muscle on the right is much further over and the breast ducts are drooping in the lower portion on the breast. This appearance can result from similar positioning errors as indicated in Figure 9.11 but in this case the difference is more extreme. The potential is for the lower portion of the breast to be blurred as compression does not hold. If this was the case the category would change from Moderate to Inadequate and require repeating.

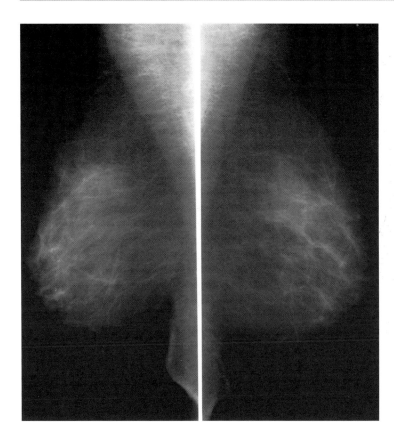

Figure 9.13 Moderate obliques. The folds at the inframammary are quite considerable. As they are extreme an air gap is present between the breast and the film holder. This has resulted in blackening of this area making diagnosis difficult without a bright light. The slight difference in the muscle position on the right has meant that the fold at the inframammary on the right is worse than on the left.

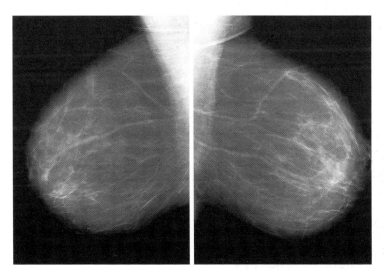

Figure 9.14 Moderate obliques. Both the films in this examination are about 2 to 3 cm too high. Tension on the muscles resulting from a film that is high will make lifting the breast difficult. When the breast is lifted against a tense and therefore rigid muscle, 'rings of Saturn' are produced. The films are very slightly asymmetrical with the left breast more stretched than the right. As a result the rings of Saturn are more marked. Again on the right there is evidence of both pectoralis major and minor, which is not evident on the left.

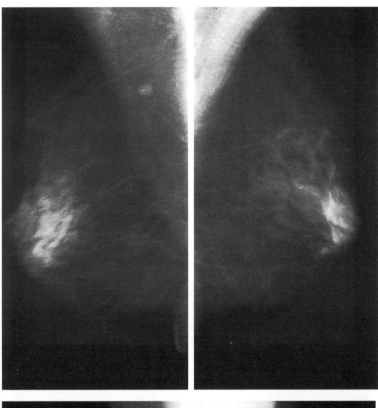

Figure 9.15 Inadequate mammograms. Apart from a series of minor faults on the right side, the left side does not demonstrate the whole breast as the muscle does not reach within 1 cm of the posterior nipple line. The left side needs to be repeated.

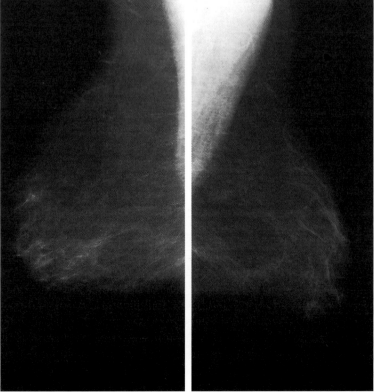

Figure 9.16 Inadequate mammograms. The right side muscle is not far enough across and the upper outer quadrant will not have been demonstrated. On the left side the arm is over too far, demonstrating the classic convex appearance and also the pectoralis major and minor. The right side will need to be repeated. The left side may need repeating if the image is blurred.

FURTHER READING AND REFERENCES

Bassett LW, Hirbawi IA, DeBruhl N, Hayes MK. Mammographic positioning: evaluation from the view box. *Radiology* 1993; **188**(3): 803–806.

Brayley N. The need for Radiographer reporting: an accident and emergency department perspective. *Radiography* **6**(4): 227–229.

College of Radiographers. *Reporting by Radiographers. A Vision Paper*. London, College of Radiographers, 1997.

Eklund G, Cardenosa G, Parsons W. Assessing the adequacy of mammographic imaging quality. *Radiology* 1994; **190**(2): 297–307.

Ionising Radiation (Medical Exposures) Regulations. HMSO, 2000. Online: *www.legislation.hmso.gov.uk/2000*

Lee L, Stickland V, Roebuck, Wilson R. *Fundamentals of Mammography*. London, WB Saunders, 1995.

McKenzie GA, Mathers SA et al. Radiographer performed general diagnostic ultrasound: current UK practice. *Radiography* 2000; **6**: 179–188.

Naylor S, Lee L, Evans A. A study to find the optimal orientation of the cranio-caudal view for screening purposes. *Clinical Radiology* 1999; **54**: 804–806.

Naylor SM, York J. An evaluation of the pectoral muscle to nipple level as a component to assess the quality of the medio-lateral oblique mammogram. *Radiography* 1999; **5**: 107–110.

NHSBSP. *A Radiographic Quality Control Manual for Mammography*. NHSBSP Publication No 21. Sheffield: NHSBSP, 1999.

NHSBSP. *Quality Assurance Guidelines for Radiographers*. NHSBSP Publication No 30. Sheffield: NHSBSP, 2000.

Paula R, Hammond S, Cooke J, Ansell. Radiographers as film readers in screening mammography. *British Journal of Radiology* 1996; **65**: 339–341.

Price R. Radiographer reporting: origins, demise and revival of plain film reporting. *Radiography* 2000; **7**(2): 105–117.

RCR Inter-professional Roles and Responsibilities in a Radiology Service. London Royal College of Radiologist RCR ref No BFCR (98), 1998.

10

Quality assurance systems

This chapter provides an outline of:

- the co-ordination of quality assurance processes into a comprehensive system,
- the quality assurance cycle: definition of objectives; identification of criteria; setting of standards; collection of information; performance monitoring,
- differing types of mammographic services with different objectives,
- organizational requirements for a quality service: internal and external quality assurance systems,
- accreditation of mammographic services.

INTRODUCTION

The effectiveness of a mammography service depends upon the outcomes and can be judged by measuring performance against stated objectives. The performance of the service as a whole is dependent on how well each of its constituent parts performs. For this reason individual quality assurance initiatives within a service should not be considered in isolation, and a system which combines and co-ordinates the individual initiatives is required.

A great deal can be learned from the experience of others and wherever possible systems should be established which facilitate comparison of quality assurance procedures between similar mammography services. This is best achieved by establishing a centrally monitored and formally organized quality assurance network. Such a set-up will tend to ensure that the overall standard of services will be high. In this way all the women who require a mammographic service can be assured that, wherever they seek that service, they can be confident that a uniformly high standard of care will be available. Such a system has been established in the National Health Service (NHS) in the UK.

TOTAL QUALITY SYSTEM

One technique frequently used to assist in the quality assurance (QA) of a whole service is total quality management (TQM). It is preferable to view this as the integration of a series of 'grass roots'-led quality processes, each designed for individual elements of a service, rather than as something imposed from above. The majority of these quality initiatives have been considered previously. In this chapter we will deal with the co-ordination of the separate elements and the integration of these into a complete QA system.

A QA system is made up of several separate elements:

- the definition of objectives,
- the identification of criteria, whereby the objectives may be measured,
- the agreement of standards,
- the collection of information,
- the review of performance,
- following the review, the definition of new objectives, the confirmation of the validity of criteria and the introduction of new criteria if required. Similarly standards should be

changed if they prove to be too lax or too ambitious.

These elements are best considered as forming a QA cycle (**Figure 10.1**). This quality assurance cycle is equally appropriate when applied to the performance of a technical process, an individual, a professional group or to a service as a whole. It can be seen, therefore, that it is a basic necessity for a service to have clearly defined objectives. These must be known to all participants in that service and those that are relevant should also be clearly stated to the users of that service.

Definition of objectives

There are two types of objectives – **outcome objectives** and **process objectives**. For instance, a screening service outcome objective could be defined as the reduction in mortality from breast cancer in the targeted population. 'En route' to this objective, each section of the service could define several different objectives relating to differing roles in the screening process. It could be the radiographer's objective to produce first-class mammograms, the radiologist's to diagnose the maximum number of small cancers, the surgeon's to achieve a low incidence of cancer recurrence, and the whole team to have a satisfied woman. These are process objectives, and each of these too has its own quality cycle.

However, both outcome and process objectives will vary according to the type of service, and essentially they are dependent upon the facilities available. The facilities should be chosen with care to ensure that the required objectives can be achieved. Facilities and objectives are unavoidably interdependent, and are considered together below, according to the differing types of service.

Identification of criteria

Criteria must be simple, meaningful and repeatable. They should represent exactly what is being measured. Importantly, they should be easily understood and easily implemented. Examples of criteria relating to process objectives defined

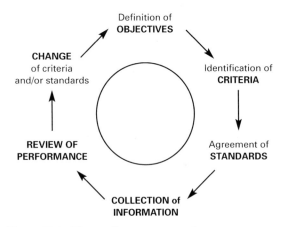

Figure 10.1 The quality assurance cycle.

for the UK National Health Service Breast Screening Programme (NHSBSP) are given in **Table 10.1**.

Agreement of standards

There are two types of standards – those that are acceptable and those that are achievable. Acceptable standards represent the minimum performance required to achieve the objectives to which they relate. Achievable standards represent the level of performance that the service should aspire to. These are standards achieved by the best 10% of services, and are of value as targets for units which are performing less well. Standards of both types should be agreed by the profession to which they relate. Examples of both acceptable and achievable standards are given in **Table 10.1**.

Table 10.1 Criteria and objectives for the UK National Health Service Breast Screening Programme.

Objective	Criteria	Acceptable standard	Achievable standard
To maximize the number of eligible women attending for screening	Proportion of eligible women who attend for screening	70% of women invited to attend for screening	75%
To maximize the number of cancers detected	The rate of cancers detected in eligible women invited and screened	>50 per 10 000 (first screen) >35 per 10 000 (repeat screens)	60 per 10 000 (first screen)
To maximize the number of small cancers detected	The proportion of invasive cancers < or = 10mm in screened women	15 in 10 000	
To achieve optimum image quality	(a) High contrast spatial resolution (b) Minimal detectable contrast (approx) 5–6 mm detail 0.5 mm detail	10 Lp/mm 1% 5%	
To limit radiation dose	Average glandular dose per film to average breast using a grid	Less than 2 mGy	
To minimize the number of women undergoing repeat films	Number of repeated examinations	Less than 3% of total Less than 2% examinations	
To minimize the number of women referred for further tests	Onward referral to Assessment	Less than 7% of women screened	5% on first screen 3% On re-screens
To minimize the number of unnecessary invasive procedures	(a) Malignant to benign biopsy ratio	1:1	1.5:1
	(b) PPV (c) Benign biopsy rate	50% <50 per 10 000 (first screen) <35 per 10 000 (repeat screens)	60% <40 per 10 000
To minimize the number of cancers in the women screened presenting between screening episodes	The proportion of cancers presenting in screened women in the subsequent 12 months	Not more than 3 per 10 000 women screened	

Collection of information

The key to an accurate and efficient quality assurance process is the availability of accurate data, without which it is impossible to monitor performance. A good, user-friendly computer system is necessary to collate and analyse these data in an efficient way.

A schedule of data collected to administer the quality assurance system in the UK breast screening programme is given in **Table 10.1**. With very few exceptions the same objectives, and therefore criteria and standards, can be adopted by units providing services for symptomatic patients. The data required to monitor the effectiveness and efficiency of a symptomatic breast imaging service are very similar to those needed for the quality assurance system of a screening service.

Review of performance

It is important that a review of performance does not become a 'witch hunt'. It should be conducted on the basis of friendly, open discussions, aimed at motivating in areas of underperformance, and congratulating in areas of achievement. In addition to group reviews, it is of great importance that individuals should review their own performance, measuring this against the approved standards and the performance of their peers (personal performance audit).

Organizational requirements

In order that the various elements within a mammographic service can function to the best possible standards, it is essential that the optimal organizational environment is provided within which they can function efficiently.

Background education

The foundation to a quality service is education. An on-going education programme is needed, not only for the medical, paramedical, administrative and clerical staff involved in delivering the service, but also for the referring personnel and the general public as potential users of the service.

A mammographic unit which has the objective to provide a high-quality service must employ staff who are fully trained in the techniques which they are required to undertake within the unit. Bad mammography is worse than no mammography. Good mammography implies mammograms which are produced by trained expert radiographers using a meticulously accurate technique, and are then interpreted by expert radiologists, fully trained and experienced in mammography. Anything less will give rise to false diagnoses of cancer, and, what is worse still, 'missing' the diagnoses of cancers which are at a small and still potentially curable stage.

In order to understand fully the part played by other professions, the personnel involved in service delivery will need an initial multidisciplinary course, followed by specific training in their own field. Refresher and update courses are also required in such a rapidly developing field as breast disease diagnosis and management.

Availability and accessibility

In the public eye the quality of a service depends on an appreciation of the reasonableness of any restrictions placed upon the woman who might attend, and the geographical accessibility of the service to that woman.

When restrictions are in force, such as age limitations for a screening service, the reasons for these should be clearly stated to the general public. Women who request a service, but are refused, should be given details of any appropriate existing alternatives which may be available. Should a woman complain of a breast problem and request an attendance at a unit which is not geared to providing the type of service she really requires, it is an essential of good practice to advise her of the action she should take, and whom she should consult.

Geographical accessibility is a major consideration, particularly in the organization of a screening service, when maximum participation is a prime objective. Local transport availability should be considered during the determination of the siting of a service. It may be preferable to serve some areas using basic mammographic apparatus installed in a mobile caravan or trailer.

Availability of assessment

It is essential that both basic and sophisticated mammographic services have rapid and easy access to an expert assessment service. When cases are referred by a generalist practitioner, either a family doctor, a general surgeon or physician, the access to an assessment service is best achieved by a pre-existing arrangement. It should be mutually agreed that should a significant abnormality be detected, then the mammographic service arranges a direct referral to a named assessment service, staffed by appropriate specialists. This entails continuing close liaison between all parties involved, including importantly, full, honest and clear communication with the woman, explaining the reasons for the assessment in terms that have been agreed by both the referring parties and the assessment personnel.

Professional organization for quality assurance

Each professional group should undertake the establishment and operation of its own QA system. This entails the definition of professional objectives, the identification of criteria whereby they can be measured, and the setting of standards. Probably the most important part of the quality cycle to be undertaken by members of a profession is the monitoring of professional performance. Not only is a profession in the best position to understand the niceties of its own practice but members of that profession are more likely to take cognisance of colleagues. If a profession does not do this then some bureaucratic organization will sooner or later undertake these responsibilities.

Internal quality assurance systems

Procedures within a unit can be controlled by an organized system such as that employed in the quality management system leading to approval under International Quality Standard ISO 9002,

European Standard EN 290002. These standards, which are all equivalent, are designed for industrial procedures but can be adapted to mammographic services with a little ingenuity. However, following a trial to evaluate the use of BS 5750 in the British screening service it was decided not to recommend its adoption on a national basis.

The units involved in the evaluation identified key benefits of the BS 5750 system as:

- the personal involvement of each individual working in the service, giving an individual appreciation of the QA procedures and of their own part in the production of a high-quality service,
- a systematic review of existing procedures to identify and change those which are not optimally efficient,
- a reporting system whereby when a procedure fails to function properly, this fact is recorded and corrective action taken.

It is considered that these beneficial aspects can be introduced into the QA system of a unit without the external auditing of the International Standard.

External quality assurance systems

In addition to self assessment, which is crucial to a satisfactory quality of performance, there should be a method to have performance assessed by an outside agency – an external quality assessment procedure. As has already been stated, it is preferable that this is organized on an individual professional basis and undertaken by members of that profession.

Radiographers in the UK screening programme have organized an accreditation system for themselves based essentially upon a full training course with periods of attachment to an active training unit. Performance is measured by the quality of the examinations performed by each radiographer being assessed by an external, appropriately qualified radiographer (see **Chapter 9**). There is a requirement to attend a number of recognized training courses each year in order to maintain accreditation.

Similarly, radiologists have a series of test films which they read on an annual basis, and pathologists a series of microscope slides which are circulated to participating personnel.

MAMMOGRAPHY SERVICE ACCREDITATION

No British mammographic service has yet undertaken the task of accreditation of individual units, but the Australian screening service and many services in the USA have an established accreditation system.

There are advantages which result from the accreditation of units within a service. These accrue to the women who use the service, those employed within the service and also to those who fund the service.

It is notoriously difficult for a woman to assess the quality of a service before she attends and commits herself to the administration of that service. An accreditation system will enable her to make a ready judgement and to avoid unaccredited units which are more likely to be substandard. Personnel working within a service are more likely to have an enhanced sense of pride should their unit be fully accredited. If a unit is being funded by an external source, then the funding authority will be anxious to ensure that its finances are being expended upon a worthwhile service.

Objectives need to be identified by the accrediting body which must be achieved before a unit is accredited. This implies the identification of appropriate criteria and standards by which these may be measured. A review of performance, measured against the agreed standards, should be undertaken at regular, usually annual, intervals.

An accredited service should:

- only employ individuals who have been fully trained in the techniques they are to perform,
- only employ individuals who regularly attend update and refresher courses,
- promulgate the process objectives defined by the accrediting body,
- give evidence that these objectives are being achieved by the submission of data of

performance measures which may be compared with the required standards. In this regard a few 'key' performance indicators can be identified,

- undertake more than the minimal workload considered by the accrediting body to be sufficient to maintain adequate expertise.

An accrediting body should have the confidence of:

- the individuals working within the service,
- the professional colleges and organizations representing the employed personnel,
- the users of the service.

Full details of the Australian and American accreditation systems may be obtained by reference to the publications listed in the Further Reading Section at the end of this chapter.

BRITISH SCREENING SERVICE QA SYSTEM

A co-ordinated, nationwide, quality assurance process has proved to be effective in the UK breast screening programme. A diagrammatic representation of the radiographers' section is

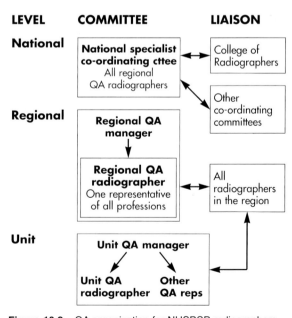

Figure 10.2 QA organization for NHSBSP radiographers.

given in **Figure 10.2**. The system comprises both internal and external aspects of QA. The UK National Health Service is administered on the basis of regions, each of which contains about eight to ten mammographic services, most of which are involved with breast cancer screening.

In the quality assurance system developed by the British screening programme, a representative of each involved profession is identified in each region. The regional representatives of each individual profession meet on a national basis, usually in association with the appropriate college or professional body. It is at these meetings that objectives are identified and standards agreed. The national level committees also review performance of the whole programme and of their own professional elements of the service in particular, with access to details of performance down to regional level. Matters concerning individual performance are not a matter for national level committees.

All the professional representatives employed within a region also meet as a multidisciplinary committee under the chairmanship of a regional QA manager. This committee has the responsibility to implement QA procedures and to monitor the performance of the region as a whole, with details of performance down to unit level. This committee also organizes regular routine visits to each individual unit by a multidisciplinary group to meet the unit personnel. The objective of these visits is to discuss, on a friendly, informal basis, matters of quality which may be brought up either by the visiting team or by the personnel of the unit visited. It has been found that such visits are of considerable value, not least in instances where a local unit is experiencing difficulties in obtaining full co-operation from the authorities in such matters as accommodation or equipment purchase.

A member of the team working within each unit is nominated as unit QA manager. This individual, usually a radiographer, has the responsibility to oversee the implementation of internal QA procedures, and to ensure participation in external QA. The unit QA manager will need considerable tact and diplomacy in dealing with the performance of sections within the unit and particularly when considering matters relating to the performance of individuals. It is the lead professional (section head) in a unit who has the prime responsibility of monitoring the performance of the other members of that profession in that section. There is consultation when necessary with the appropriate regional professional representative. In undertaking this responsibility, a close liaison must be maintained between the section head and the unit QA manager, without prejudicing professional relationships.

There is a full series of booklets produced for the UK NHSBSP by the various professional groups, which detail the QA processes to be adopted by each profession.

The National Breast Screening programme has produced a Systematic Management Programme for use in all screening services. This has many of the features of the International Standard.

FURTHER READING

British Standard Institution. *British Standard Quality Systems. Part 2 Specification for Production and Installation*. BS 5750. London: BSI, 1987.

DeBruhl ND, Farria DM, Bassett LW. Strategies for implementation and quality assurance for mammographic screening. *Current Opinion in Radiology* 1992; **4**: 155–159.

Europe Against Cancer Study Group. *European Guidelines for Quality Assurance in Mammography Screening*. Nijmegen, Netherlands: LRCB/KUN, 1992.

European Committee for Standardisation. *Quality Systems – Model for Quality Assurance in Production and Installation. EN 29002*. Brussels: CEN B-1000, 1987.

Farria DM, Bassett LW, Kimme-Smith C, DeBruhl N. Mammographic quality assurance from A to Z. *Radiographics* 1994; **14**: 371–385.

Gray JAM. *General Principles of Quality Assurance in Breast Cancer Screening*. Oxford: NHSBSP Publications, 1989.

Guyer PB, Dewbury KC. In: *Sonomammography – An Atlas of Comparative Breast Ultrasound*. Chichester: John Wiley, 1987; 2–3.

Hendrick RE. Quality assurance in mammography: accreditation, legislation and compliance with quality assurance standards. *Radiological Clinics of North America* 1992; **30**: 234–256.

Hendrick RE, Haus AG, Hubbard LB et al. American College of Radiology accreditation program for mammographic screening sites: physical evaluation criteria. *Radiology* 1987; **165(P)**: 209.

International Organisation for Standardisation. *Quality Systems – Model for Quality Assurance in Production and Installation. ISO 9002–1987*.

McLelland R, Hendrick RE, Zinninger MD, Wilcox PA. The American College of Radiology mammography accreditation program. *American Journal of Roentgenology* 1991; **157**: 473–479.

National Advisory Committee for the Early Detection of Breast Cancer Working Party. *National Accreditation Guidelines*. Canberra: Department of Health Housing and Community Services, ACT 2601, 1992.

National Co-ordinating Group for Surgeons. *Quality Assurance Guidelines for Surgeons in Breast Cancer Screening*. NHSBSP Publication No. 20. Sheffield: NHSBSP, 1992.

National Council on Radiation Protection and Measurements. *Mammography – a User's Guide*. NRCP Report No. 85. Bethesda, MD: NRCP, 1986.

NHSBSP Radiographers Quality Assurance Co-ordination Committee. *Quality Assurance Guidelines for Radiographers*. NHSBSP Publication No. 30. Sheffield: NHSBSP, 2000.

NHSBSP Systematic Management of Quality for Breast Screening Units. NHSBSP publication No 34, Part II. NHSBSP, Sheffield, 1999.

Patnick J, Gray JAM. *Guidelines on the Collection and use of Breast Cancer Data*. NHSBSP Publication No. 26. Sheffield: NHSBSP, 1993.

Pritchard J, ed. *Quality Assurance Guidelines for Mammography*. Report of a Sub-committee of the Radiology Advisory Committee of the Chief Medical Officer. Oxford: NHSBSP Publications, 1989.

Royal Australasian College of Radiologists. Accreditation guidelines for screening mammographic facilities. *RACR Newsletter* 1990; **29**: 19–21.

Royal College of Radiologists. *Quality Assurance Guidelines for Radiologists*. Oxford: NHSBSP Publications, 1990.

Shoderu B, Langham S, Normand C. *The Pilot Registration of the Epping Breast Screening Service under BS5750 – an Economic Evaluation*. Department of Public Health & Policy – Health Services Research Unit. London: London School of Hygiene & Tropical Medicine, 1992.

11

The basis of mammographic interpretation

This chapter provides an outline of:

- the role of mammography in breast cancer diagnosis,
- common variants of normality,
- common benign conditions,
- histological types of breast cancer,
- the likelihood of radiographic signs being due to benign or malignant disease: mass lesions, spiculate lesions, architectural distortion, calcifications.

INTRODUCTION

This chapter describes common abnormalities that affect the breast. An understanding of the mammographic features of breast conditions will help the radiographer to perform good-quality mammograms.

THE ROLE OF MAMMOGRAPHY

The role of mammography varies according to the reason for a woman's examination. Mammography may demonstrate an unsuspected abnormality as a result of screening or may be used in the assessment of women with symptoms. In both these instances its role is to exclude or confirm a malignant process. When employed in conjunction with clinical assessment and cytology/histopathology, a definitive diagnosis of benign disease may be obtained and the patient saved unnecessary surgical intervention.

The role of mammography in the assessment of women with symptoms which suggest benign problems is to confirm benignity and exclude a malignant process. There are only a few localized benign problems that can be diagnosed with certainty on mammography. Ultrasound of the breast is a useful adjunct to mammography in these circumstances, with differentiation of cystic from solid lesions and characterization of solid lesions being of particular clinical value.

The role of mammography in the assessment of malignant disease of the breast is more complex and better defined. Mammography will demonstrate the majority of palpable breast tumours and will almost always show signs helpful in differentiating benign from malignant processes. Mammography may also detect malignancy well before it is the cause of clinical signs or symptoms. On average, mammography will detect breast cancer 2 years before it causes signs or symptoms. This is why mammography is effective in screening for breast cancer. However, not all breast cancers, even when clearly palpable, are visible on mammography. There are a variety of reasons for this. Some breasts are very dense on mammography, to such an extent that even large lesions are not discernible within the dense normal tissues. In other cases the breast cancer is of a type that does not disrupt or disturb the normal breast architecture and hence is invisible on mammography.

There is excellent correlation between the imaging and histopathological findings of breast carcinoma and imaging plays a fundamental role in the diagnosis and treatment of malignant disease. Mammography is more accurate than palpation in assessing the size of a tumour, will show the extent of the disease by detecting multifocal disease, may show associated ductal carcinoma in situ, and will confirm that the opposite breast is disease-free. Knowledge of all these factors is essential to the proper management of breast cancer.

Indications for mammography

Mammography is rarely indicated in young women. Almost all breast symptoms in young women are caused by benign or physiological processes and mammography has little to offer in their management. Breast cancer is very rare under the age of 30 and is uncommon under the age of 35. The young breast is inclined to be denser on mammography and lesions are less likely to be visible. The young breast is theoretically more susceptible to the carcinogenic effects of ionizing radiation, although the risks of cancer induction by mammography are small at any age. These factors mean that mammography is rarely indicated in the assessment of symptoms in women under 35 years of age unless there is a strong clinical indication of malignancy. The increasing frequency of breast cancer as a possible cause of symptoms justifies the use of mammography in women over 35 years with significant breast symptoms. In the absence of symptoms mammography cannot be justified as a screening tool in women under the age of 40. Mammographic screening is of proven value in women aged 40–70. The main reason for few programmes screening women aged 40–49 is poor cost effectiveness. Women under 50 with a strong family history may benefit from screening. Women over 50 who present with breast symptoms probably all deserve a mammogram as part of their clinical assessment.

Ultrasound should be the imaging technique of first choice in younger women and is useful in the further assessment of lesions demonstrated on mammography. Ultrasound is not an effective technique for screening for breast cancer at any age.

The influence of age and hormone replacement therapy on mammographic sensitivity

The density of the breast on mammography does vary with age, with younger premenopausal women more likely to show a dense background pattern (**Figure 11.1**). The denser the breast the more likely it is that subtle mammographic signs will be obscured. It is therefore not surprising that breast cancers are not always visible on a mammogram, even when clinically palpable, and that this is more likely to be the case in younger women. Hormone replacement therapy causes an increase in mammographic density in many women. This leads to a decrease in the

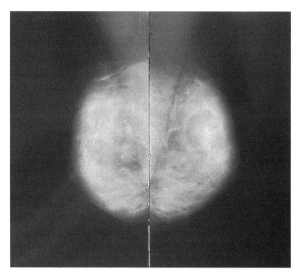

Figure 11.1 Bilateral medio-lateral oblique mammograms showing a homogenously dense background pattern.

sensitivity of screening mammography of 7–21%.

BENIGN BREAST CONDITIONS

Benign breast changes

The normal monthly variations of female sex hormones have an effect in the breast leading to a large variety of findings histologically and radiologically. These variations are normal, often bilateral and symmetrical, and usually symptomless. Collectively these changes are commonly referred to as benign breast changes (BBC) or as aberrations of normal development and involution (ANDI). In the past numerous names have been used to describe the various entities within this group of conditions – chronic mastitis, cystic mastitis, mastopathy, fibroadenosis and mazoplasia being amongst the more common. In the absence of evidence of any disease process, some considered it better to discard the term disease completely. Since this whole group of conditions can be simply explained on the basis of variations of normal processes it is now common practice to call them collectively 'benign breast changes'.

These changes are the principal cause of the various different normal background patterns found on mammography of normal women. The

major types of background were described by Wolfe (1967) as parenchymal pattern types P1, P2 and DY, with type N1 being an absence of the others. His classification is still widely adopted, even though the initial impression that there was an increase in the risk of developing breast cancer associated with the DY and P2 types has since been shown to be greatly exaggerated.

The mammographic appearances vary according to the structures which are mainly affected. The two most commonly involved are the larger ducts and the terminal duct lobular units (TDLs).

Fibroadenomatoid hyperplasia

Fibroadenomatoid hyperplasia is a condition showing mixed features of fibrocystic change and fibroadenoma. It is a common cause of indeterminate mammographic calcification. Diagnosis is readily confirmed by image-guided core biopsy (**Figure 11.2**).

Duct ectasia

Occasionally dilated ducts can become filled with debris which may calcify, a feature that is

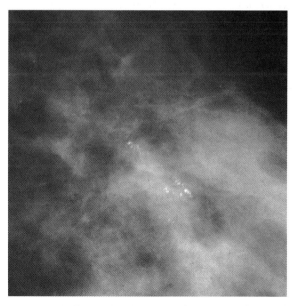

Figure 11.2 Mammographic image showing a pleomorphic cluster of granular microcalcifications. Histologically this was shown to be fibroadenomatoid hyperplasia.

often visible on a mammogram (broken needle appearance). Duct contents may escape into the surrounding tissue, exciting an inflammatory reaction (periductal mastitis). On occasions the end result of this process can be visualized on a mammogram as small calcified plates surrounding and running alongside the ducts, giving a characteristic 'pipe stem' appearance (**Figure 11.3**). Calcifications are the most common mammographic manifestation of duct ectasia.

Cyst formation

Cystic changes in the breast are very common. During normal cyclical activity the cells lining the TDLs increase in size and an increase in the diameter of the lobules is often seen associated with this. On occasions this dilatation is to such a degree that cysts are formed. Any condition in which the rate of secretion by the epithelial cells exceeds the capacity of the duct to drain the lobule, will cause the lobule to dilate and a cyst will form. Some cysts may dilate to a size which renders them visible on imaging either by mam-

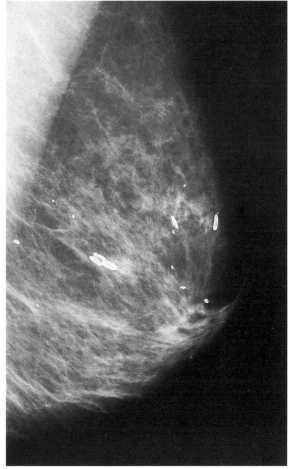

(b)

Figure 11.3b　Mammographic image showing periductal fat necrosis. This appearance is sometimes called a 'pipe stem' appearance.

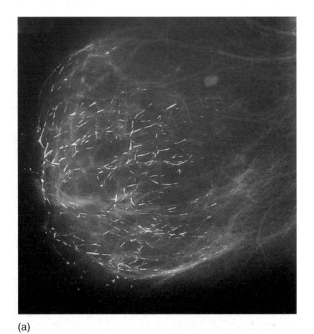

(a)

Figure 11.3a　Mammographic image showing extensive intraductal calcification. This is due to duct ectasia. This is sometimes described as a broken needle appearance.

mography or ultrasound (**Figure 11.4**). A few of them may dilate further and become palpable. Should one or two cysts be palpable within a breast then it is highly likely that more will be demonstrated by mammography or ultrasound.

An inflammatory reaction may also occur around dilated TDLs and lead to fibrosis. The combination of fibrosis and cyst formation is known as fibrocystic change. This may be visualized on a mammogram as an increase in density, or on ultrasound examination as a diffuse increase in small echoes in the affected region, together with cysts of various sizes.

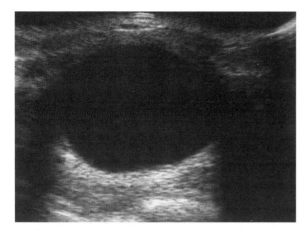

Figure 11.4 Ultrasound image showing a transonic rounded structure with distal bright up and edge attenuation. The appearances are those of a simple cyst.

Cyst contents often have a high concentration of calcium which may precipitate to form minute dust-like particles suspended in the cyst fluid. This is known as milk of calcium. The calcium particles sink to the bottom of the cyst and, when viewed on a projection taken with a vertical beam, the collection of calcific particles will be seen as a soft density with a rounded margin.

When viewed on a projection using a horizontal x-ray beam the density will be crescentic, having a straight upper margin. This appearance is known as the 'tea cup' sign, and is characteristic and diagnostic of fibrocystic change (**Figure 11.5**).

Sclerosing lesions

Another lesion which may give rise to mammographic features is the radial scar. The central part of the lesion shows fibrosis which contracts to form a scar which causes distortion of the normal surrounding architecture. Calcifications are a commonly associated feature. Typically the lesions are discoid in shape, and are therefore more easily visible 'en face' than if projected end on. This may result in a radial scar being more clearly visible in one projection than another. On mammography the deformity caused by a radial scar is indistinguishable from that caused by a carcinoma (**Figure 11.6**). Screening mammography will detect about two radial scars in every 1000 women screened.

If a large area is involved in this sclerosing, deforming process then the condition is called a complex sclerosing lesion. The mass of tissue so

Figure 11.5 Lateral magnification view of calcifications showing the 'tea cup' sign which is characteristic of fibrocystic change.

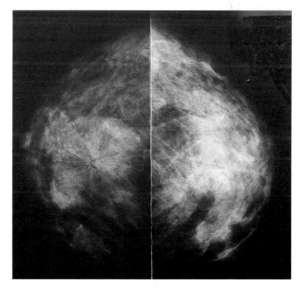

Figure 11.6 Bilateral CC views showing an area of parenchymal distortion centrally within the right breast. This was shown to be a radial scar.

formed may feel hard and fixed to the surrounding tissues on palpation and can therefore be mistaken for a carcinoma. Papillary lesions which arise within breast duct are benign mass lesions which can also undergo sclerosis. Benign radial scars and papillary lesions are occasionally associated with either ductal carcinoma in situ, or even invasive cancer. For this reason, radial scars and papillary lesions are excised when diagnosed.

Another common sclerosing lesion of the breast is sclerosing adenosis. The mammographic features of sclerosing adenosis are varied and include ill-defined mass, architectural distortion and suspicious microcalcification. Sclerosing adenosis can be confirmed histologically using image-guided core biopsy.

Fibroadenoma

Proliferation of both the epithelial and stromal elements of the TDL can give rise to a localized well defined mass known as a fibroadenoma. These masses are often too small to give symptoms and may be detected as incidental findings on mammography performed for other reasons. Fibroadenomas that grow large enough to produce a palpable lump most commonly occur in women in their twenties and thirties. They are well defined, ovoid lesions of rubbery consistency. New fibroadenomas do not appear, nor are existing ones seen to grow in size, in postmenopausal women, except in women who are having hormonal replacement therapy (HRT).

On mammography a fibroadenoma is seen as a mass which displaces the normal tissues, has a smooth, rounded, well defined margin, but no specific characteristic features (**Figure 11.7**). Calcification commonly occurs in fibroadenomata, particularly in those which have been present for some time. When calcification does occur, then it often has an absolutely characteristic 'popcorn' appearance on mammography (**Figure 11.8**).

Ultrasound of fibroadenomas usually shows a well defined, oval, homogeneous, hypoechoic mass with either no distal effect or distal bright up (**Figure 11.9**).

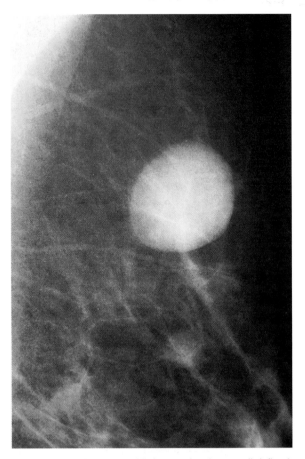

Figure 11.7 Mammographic image showing a well defined round mass. It has a smooth margin but no other characteristic features. Histologically this was fibroadenoma.

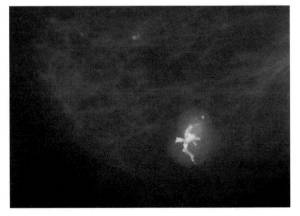

Figure 11.8 Mammographic image showing characteristic popcorn calcification within a hylanised fibroadenoma.

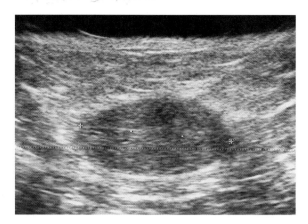

Figure 11.9 Ultrasound image of fibroadenoma. There is a well defined homogeneous mass with a round shape. There is distal acoustic bright up and the lesion is wider than it is tall.

MALIGNANT AND POTENTIALLY MALIGNANT CONDITIONS

What is breast cancer?

Cancer and carcinoma are terms used to describe uncontrolled overgrowth of abnormal cells, a disease process which may ultimately threaten the life of the host. Breast carcinoma is a term used collectively to describe a heterogeneous group of malignant conditions, the vast majority of which arise in the epithelial cells in the terminal duct lobular unit. Breast cancer can be divided into two main types – in situ carcinoma, which is contained within the ducts or lobules, and invasive carcinoma, which has spread out of the ducts or lobules through the basement membrane into the adjacent breast tissue. Invasive carcinoma has the potential to spread via the bloodstream or lymphatic vessels to other parts of the body (metastatic breast carcinoma). In situ carcinoma does not threaten life but it has the potential to become invasive and then to do so.

There are also a number of conditions that are recognized to be precancerous (**Table 11.1**). They range from those with very little risk of progression to malignancy to those with a highly significant risk. These conditions, except for DCIS, have no clearly recognizable features on mammography to distinguish them from the benign processes already described. Mammography has

Table 11.1   Histological terms used to describe the transition from normal epithelium to malignancy

Histology term	Increasing risk of developing invasive carcinoma
Normal epithelial hyperplasia (ductal and lobular) Atypical lobular hyperplasia Atypical ductal hyperplasia Lobular carcinoma in situ Ductal carcinoma in situ	↓

a very limited role in the assessment and management of these potentially malignant conditions.

Types of breast cancer

A simple classification of both in situ and invasive breast cancer is shown in **Table 11.2**. Lobular carcinoma in situ (LCIS) has no identifiable features on mammography and is almost always an incidental finding in a biopsy carried out for another reason. LCIS is a risk factor for breast cancer in either breast. By contrast, ductal carcinoma in situ (DCIS) frequently shows characteristic mammographic features, the most common of which is microcalcification. Invasive cancers usually arise directly from an area of DCIS.

Table 11.2   Pathological classification of carcinoma of the breast

A Ductal
in situ (DCIS)
Invasive

B Lobular
in situ (LCIS)
Invasive

C Medullary

D Special types
Tubular
Papillary
Mucinous
Invasive cribriform

E Mixed

F Rare types
Spindle cell
Metaplastic
Apocrine
Secretory
Inflammatory

Table 11.3 Pathological subtypes comparing screening and symptomatic presentation (cases presenting in Nottingham in 1993)

	Screening	Symptomatic
Ductal in situ	17	5
Ductal NST	30	50
Lobular	11	16
Medullary	<1	3
Mucinous	<1	1
Tubular/cribriform	15	4
Tubular mixed	20	14
Other	6	7

Numbers are percentages.

The proportion of the different types of breast cancer detected at screening differs from that seen in women of the same age with symptomatic breast cancer (**Table 11.3**). Subtypes which carry a better prognosis, sometimes referred to as special types, are more likely to be found by screening. This is for two reasons: first, screening mammography detects breast cancer at an earlier stage and, second, special-type tumours often produce features that are easier to detect on mammography.

Invasive cancer grade

The grading of invasive breast cancer is determined by the number of tubules, the number of mitoses and the degree of nuclear pleomorphism demonstrated histologically. Tumours with a low degree of nuclear pleomorphism and low counts of mitoses and high counts of tubule formation are low-grade tumours. Tumours with no tubule formation, high in miototic counts and a high degree of pleomorphism are high grade. The histological grade of an invasive cancer is the major intrinsic prognostic factor. High-grade tumours carry a poor prognosis where low-grade tumours carry a good prognosis. Cancers detected by mammographic screening are on average of a lower histological grade than cancers presenting symptomatically. Mammographically high-grade invasive cancers present as either an ill-defined or spiculate mass which is commonly associated with casting-type calcification. Low-grade invasive cancers normally present as a small spiculate mass or architectural distortion and calcification is much less common.

THE MAMMOGRAPHIC FEATURES OF BREAST CANCER ACCORDING TO PATHOLOGICAL TYPES

Ductal carcinoma in situ (DCIS)

DCIS accounts for around 15–20% of screen-detected cancers compared to 5% of symptomatic cancers. In the 40–50 years age band it may account for 40% of all screen-detected cancers. This is because DCIS rarely gives rise to clinical symptoms, while its primary mammographic sign, microcalcification, is easy to detect at a preclinical stage. DCIS may be broadly divided into two types, high-grade and low-grade, both of which are most commonly seen as microcalcification.

The microcalcifications typical of high-grade DCIS (casts, branching and granular microcalcifications in a ductal distribution) are produced by calcification of necrotic tissue in the centre of the affected ducts (**Figure 11.10**). The extent of mammographic microcalcification in high-grade DCIS correlates well with the actual extent of the disease. High-grade DCIS is an aggressive

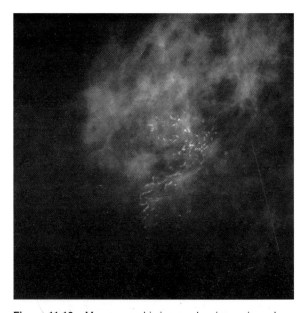

Figure 11.10 Mammographic image showing an irregular-shaped cluster of microcalcifications. The calcifications themselves show marked pleomorphism and a ductal distribution. The appearances are those of high-grade ductal carcinoma in situ.

process with 30–50% of cases progressing to invasive carcinoma within 5 years. Paget's disease of the nipple, which usually presents as nipple inflammation similar to eczema, is a form of DCIS.

The microcalcifications associated with low-grade DCIS tend to be better defined and form as pearl-like laminated structures within the mucin-containing intercellular spaces. These calcifications may be morphologically indistinguishable from those associated with benign breast change. They are therefore more difficult to recognize as malignant, their distribution being the most important feature. Malignant microcalcifications tend to be arranged in linear, irregular or V-shaped clusters, while benign microcalcifications tend to be arranged in rounded clusters. Low-grade DCIS has a risk of invasion of 40% at 30 years follow up.

DCIS is also an important feature to document in association with invasive carcinoma as its presence often means breast conservation surgery is not appropriate. Breast-conserving treatment for DCIS requires careful preoperative evaluation, in which mammography plays a very important role. Knowledge of the mammographic spectrum of DCIS is essential for this process.

Invasive ductal carcinoma

Invasive ductal carcinoma is the commonest histological type of breast cancer and is often referred to as ductal carcinoma of no specific type (ductal NST). It has a wide spectrum of appearances on mammography, but the commonest is spiculate mass. Other less common mammographic features are ill-defined irregular mass, parenchymal distortion, asymmetry and calcification. The parenchymal distortion is caused by the fibrous reaction causing pulling in of adjacent structures.

Approximately a third of invasive ductal carcinomas are associated with microcalcification. The combination of a spiculate mass and microcalcification is very strong evidence of malignancy.

Lobular carcinoma in situ (LCIS)

LCIS has no specific mammographic features. It is not a true malignancy and should be regarded simply as a risk factor. LCIS itself rarely calcifies but is often associated with benign processes which produce microcalcification. LCIS is usually an incidental finding in biopsy specimens.

Invasive lobular carcinoma

Invasive lobular carcinoma cannot be distinguished from ductal carcinoma by its mammographic appearances. The majority of lobular carcinomas show very similar features to ductal carcinoma, with a spiculate mass being the most common appearance, but a few produce little or no mammographic abnormality despite being large in size. Microcalcification is less commonly seen in association with lobular carcinoma.

Medullary carcinoma

Medullary carcinoma is rare. It is most often demonstrated as a partly well defined, dense mass lesion without architectural distortion (**Figure 11.11**). As such it may mimic a benign lesion such as a cyst or fibroadenoma.

Mucinous carcinoma

Mucinous carcinoma is another uncommon tumour which also produces a partly well

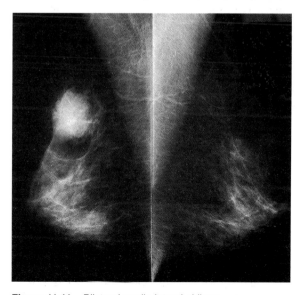

Figure 11.11 Bilateral medio-lateral oblique mammography showing a predominantly ill-defined mass in the upper right breast. Histologically this was shown to be a medullary carcinoma.

defined mass on mammography. Its mucinous content can result in distal enhancement on ultrasound, a feature usually associated with benign lesions.

Tubular carcinoma

Tubular carcinoma is found much more commonly as a result of screening (**Table 11.3**). Tubular carcinoma typically produces architectural distortion which is more extensive than would be expected for the size of the central tumour mass. This feature is easy to detect on mammography and, as a result, many can be detected at a small size. Tubular carcinomas often have features that are indistinguishable on mammography from radial scar or complex sclerosing lesions. Some carcinomas have features of more than one tumour type. The commonest of such lesions are tubular mixed cancers with features and prognosis intermediate between these of tubular cancer and ductal carcinomas of no specific type.

MAMMOGRAPHIC FEATURES OF MALIGNANCY

No mammographic feature can indicate that a particular lesion is benign or malignant with certainty. Some features may be highly suggestive of a benign diagnosis while others are typical of malignancy (**Table 11.4**). However, many mammographic signs are less clear cut and the differentiation of benign and malignant conditions requires further imaging, clinical assessment and cytological/histological examinations.

Table 11.4 The positive predictive value (PPV) of mammographic features for malignancy (Nottingham, 1993)

	PPV of malignancy (%)
Well circumscribed mass	<1
Ill-defined mass	50
Spiculate mass lesion	>95
Parenchymal deformity	40
Asymmetries	<1
Suspicious microcalcification	40

There are four primary mammographic features that may indicate the presence of a breast abnormality:

- mass,
- parenchymal deformity,
- asymmetric density,
- microcalcifications.

Mass

A mass is defined as a central area of increased density with generally convex margins. Masses can be divided into those that are well defined, poorly defined or spiculate (**Table 11.5 and Figures 11.12, 11.13 and 11.14**). A well defined mass, particularly if it shows a 'halo' on mammography, is very likely to be benign whatever its size. Age is an important factor in the differential diagnosis of a well defined mass. Under the age of 35 a fibroadenoma is the most likely diagnosis. Between 35 and 55 cysts are very common. After 55 the vast majority of well defined masses are still benign but a well circumscribed carcinoma becomes a credible possibility. Lobulation is suggestive of benignity. Masses which appear ill-defined in any part of their margin on mammography must be considered suspicious and always require further assessment. Ultrasound is ideal for distinguishing cysts from solid lesions. Ultrasound is also useful in differentiating benign from malignant masses. Malignant masses on ultrasound are usually

Table 11.5 Differential diagnosis of masses demonstrated on mammography

Well defined mass	Poorly defined mass	Spiculate Mass
Cyst	Carcinoma	Carcinoma
Fibroadenoma	Haematoma	Complex sclerosing lesion
Lymph node	Fat-necrosis	Surgical scar
Papilloma	Abscess	
Sebaceous cyst	Fibroadenoma	
Abscess		
Haematoma		
Hamartoma		

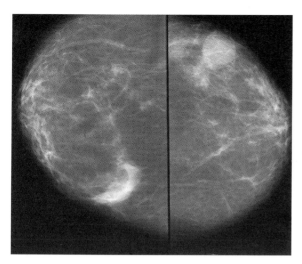

Figure 11.12 Bilateral CC views showing a low-density well defined mass in the lateral left breast. The appearance is of a benign lesion such as cyst or fibroadenoma. Such an appearance has a less than 1% chance of being due to malignancy.

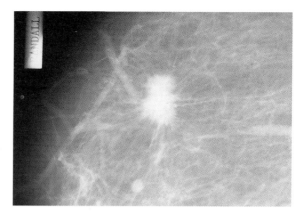

Figure 11.14 Localized mammographic image showing a spiculated mass. Such an appearance has a very high chance of being due to invasive carcinoma.

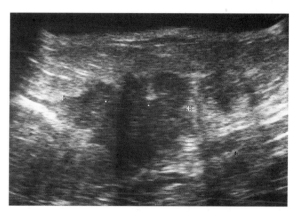

Figure 11.15 Ultrasound image showing a malignant mass. The mass is ill-defined and has an irregular outline. There is irregular posterior attenuation and intraductal extension of the tumour is demonstrated to the left side of the image.

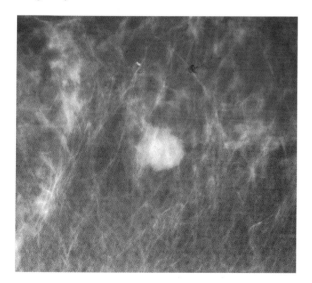

Figure 11.13 Localized mammographic view showing an ill-defined mass. Although such a mass may be due to a cyst or fibroadenoma with surrounding fibrosis, there is an approximately 30% chance of this mass being due to a carcinoma.

inhomogeneous, poorly defined masses with distal shadowing which are often taller than they are wide (**Figure 11.15**). Ultrasound is also useful in defining the extent of malignant lesions.

A spiculate mass is defined as an irregular mass with ill-defined margins and surrounding parenchymal reaction, producing spicules and tentacles (representing a combination of pulling in of surrounding fibrous bands and outgrowths of the cancer into the surrounding breast). Spiculate lesions should always be considered malignant until proven otherwise.

Architectural distortion

Architectural distortion is defined as distortion of the normal breast parenchymal pattern. It is commonly seen in association with an ill-defined mass lesion, an appearance strongly suspicious of an invasive breast carcinoma. Architectural distortion may also occur on its own when its cause may be equally sinister.

On mammography, apparent deformity is often produced by the summation of normal overlapping shadows.

The differential diagnosis of architectural distortion without an associated mass lies between a radial scar (complex sclerosing lesion) and carcinoma. The presence or absence of associated microcalcification does not alter this differential.

Asymmetry

Asymmetry is a non-specific sign (**Figure 11.16**).

Asymmetry is common and is rarely the sole sign of malignancy. The large majority of asymmetrical densities simply represent normal breast tissue (asymmetrical involution). Asymmetry of density is defined as 'a focal area of increased density, often interspersed with varying amounts of fatty tissue and often demonstrating concave margins'. In the absence of any clinical finding, asymmetry without any other associated mammographic features is very unlikely to be of significance.

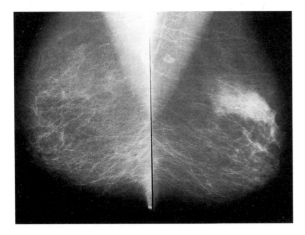

Figure 11.16 Mammographic image showing a large asymmetric density in the upper left breast. Such an appearance without additional mammographic features has a very low chance of representing malignancy and is almost always a benign/normal finding.

Microcalcifications

The majority of microcalcifications in the breast are associated with benign breast conditions (e.g. sclerosing adenosis, fibrocystic change, duct ectasia). To select the microcalcifications that represent malignant disease is not an easy task. A careful analysis of the mammographic appearances may allow microcalcifications to be divided into benign and high-risk of malignancy groups. These features include morphology, density, distribution and change with magnification and change with time (**Table 11.6**).

Round and ring calcifications are almost always benign. Granular and casting microcalcifications in a ductal distribution are much more suspicious. Clusters of calcifications are more likely to signify malignancy, whereas widespread, scattered particles are more likely to be associated with benign changes. The number of calcifications within a cluster is of no value in differential diagnosis, but the shape of a cluster can be of help. A spherical or oval cluster is likely to be benign, but any other shape is suggestive of malignancy. The only occasion when numbers of calcifications may assist in the differentiation of benign from malignant disease is following magnification. Should magnification reveal an increase in the number of calcific particles within the area of previously seen calcifications, then the chance of malignancy is increased. If extra calcifications are visualized outside the area, then the chances of malignancy are lessened. Should there be no increase in the number of particles visible, then benign disease is likely to be the cause.

Table 11.6 Features helpful in defining the cause of microcalcifications

Feature	Benign	Malignant
Cluster shape	Round	Irregular
Particle size	Large	Small
Particle shape	Round	Irregular (rods and branches)
Particle density	Low	Dense or mixed
Number on magnification	Same or widely distributed	More in cluster

SUMMARY

The following are some general observations about mammographic interpretation.

- Well defined masses are very likely to be benign.
- Ill-defined masses deserve careful assessment.
- Spiculate masses and focal areas of architectural distortion should be regarded as malignant until proven otherwise.
- Asymmetries are rarely important.

- Microcalcifications are often difficult to evaluate and may represent DCIS with or without an invasive focus.
- A spiculate mass with pleomorphic microcalcification is highly suspicious of malignancy.

The secret of success in the diagnosis of breast problems is careful clinical and imaging assessment with judicious use of core biopsy. Assessment should not stop until a definitive outcome is obtained.

REFERENCES AND FURTHER READING

Bjurstam N, Bjorneld L, Duffy SW, et al. The Gothenburg Breast Screening Trial. First results on mortality, incidence and mode of detection for women ages 39–49 years at randomization. *Cancer* 1997; **80**: 2091–2099.

Ciatto S, Rosselli Del Turco M, Catarzi S, Morrone D. The contribution of ultrasonography to the differential diagnosis of breast cancer. *Neoplasma* 1994; **41**: 341–345.

Cyrlak D, Wong CH. Mammographic changes in post menopausal women undergoing hormone replacement therapy. *American Journal of Rentgenology* 1993; **161**: 1177–1183.

Lister D, Evans AJ, Burrell HC, Blamey RW, Wilson ARM, Pinder SE, Ellis IO, Elston CW, Kollias J. The accuracy of breast ultrasound in the evaluation of clinically benign descrete, symptomatic breast lumps. *Clinical Radiology* 1998; **53**: 490–492.

Litherland JC, Stallard S, Hole D, Cordiner C. The effect of hormone replacement therapy on the sensitivity of screening mammograms. *Clinical Radiology* 1999; **54**: 285–288.

Malmo Mammographic Screening Program. Reduced breast cancer mortality in women under age 50: Updated results from the Malmo mammographic screening program. *JNCI Monograph* 1997; **22**: 63–68.

Perre CI, Koot VCM, de Hooge P, Leguit P. The value of ultrasound in the evaluation of palpable breast tumours: a prospective study of 400 cases. *European Journal of Surgical Oncology* 1994; **20**: 637–640.

Rosenberg RD, Hunt WC, Williamson MR, et al. Effects of age, breast density, ethnicity, and estrogen replacement therapy on screening mammographic sensitivity and cancer stage at diagnosis: review of 183,134 screening mammograms in Albuqueque, New Mexico. *Radiology* 1998; **209**: 511–518.

Sibbering D, Burrell H, Evans A, et al. Mammographic sensitivity in women under 50 presenting symptomatically with breast cancer. *The Breast* 1995; **4**: 127–129.

Spencer NJB, Evans AJ, Galea M, Sibbering DM, Yeoman LJ, Pinder S, Ellis IO, Elston CW, Blamey RW, Robertson JFR, Wilson ARM. Pathological-radiological correlations in benign lesions excised during a breast screening programme. *Clinical Radiology* 1994; **49**: 853–856.

Stavros AT, Thickman D, Rapp CL, Dennis MA, Parker SH, Sisney GA. Solid breast nodules: use of sonography to distinguish between benign and malignant lesions. *Radiology* 1995; **196**: 123–134.

Wald N, Murphy P, Major P, Parkes C, Townsend J, Frost C. UKCCCR multicentre randomised controlled trial of one and two view mammography in breast cancer screening. *British Medical Journal* 1995; **311**: 1189–1193.

12

Breast screening

This chapter outlines:

- breast screening has been shown to reduce breast cancer in women aged 40–69,
- screening should be by 2-view mammography alone,
- double reading with arbitration should occur,
- multidisciplinary assessment of screen-detected abnormalities is required.

INTRODUCTION

Principles of screening

Before screening for any disease becomes clinical practice it is important that a number of questions be addressed to confirm that screening will be effective. The most important questions are:

- Is the disease an important health problem for this population?
- Can the at-risk population be identified?
- Can the screening modality detect the disease at early pre-clinical stage?
- Is the screening modality acceptable to the population?
- Does early treatment lead to a better outcome?
- Is treatment of pre-clinical disease widely available?
- Are the benefits of screening larger than the harm caused?
- Is screening cost effective in comparison with other health care measures?

If the answer to all these questions is yes then screening should proceed. In this chapter on screening for breast cancer we will look at methods of screening, who to screen, when to screen and how to screen. While answering these questions it will be seen that for mammographic screening the answer to all the above questions is yes.

Epidemiology of breast cancer

Breast cancer is common in Western Europe and North America and is becoming commoner in countries adopting a Western life style. Breast cancer is the commonest cancer in women in the UK and accounts for 18% of all female cancer deaths. A total of 15,000 women die of breast cancer every year in England and Wales. These facts confirm that breast cancer is an important health problem.

The only risk factors for breast cancer which are strong enough to define a screening population are age and being female. Breast cancer becomes steadily more common with increasing age. A few women with a strong family history are also at increased risk but the efficacy of screening in this group has not been unequivocally proven.

METHODS OF SCREENING
Clinical examination

One of the first trials showing a mortality benefit for breast screening (Shapiro et al 1988) used clinical examination as well as mammography; more recent trials, which have shown an equal or greater mortality benefit, have used mammography only (Nystrom et al 1993, Bjurstam et al 1997). It has been shown that clinical examination alone cannot reduce population breast cancer mortality. The many benign abnormalities detected by clinical examination are a major disadvantage of this screening modality.

Breast self-examination

A UK population screening trial using instruction in breast self examination as the screening method showed better prognostic features in the study group but a significant mortality reduction was not seen (RR 1.01, 95% CI 0.86–1.17) (Ellman

et al 1993). However, many encourage breast self-examination in women over 30 years of age.

Mammography

Mammography has been the screening modality used for every randomized-controlled trial that has shown a significant population breast cancer mortality reduction (Shapiro et al 1988, Nystrom et al 1993, Bjurstam et al 1997). Mammography is not an ideal screening test. It is difficult to perform and interpret and some women find the procedure uncomfortable. Re-attendance rates for screening examinations are high (> 90%) indicating that the discomfort of mammography does not discourage women from attending. Mammography uses ionizing radiation and so is theoretically capable of inducing breast cancer. However this is likely to be only of practical concern in women under 35 years of age. In women of screening age (>40), the risk of inducing a breast cancer is about 1 in 100,000 examinations. While the life time risk of women in the Western world is around 1 in 12.

Mammography is a sensitive screening tool for the detection of invasive breast cancer and DCIS. However mammography is non-specific as only 1 in 5 to 1 in 10 women recalled from screening has cancer. Multidisciplinary assessment using additional imaging, clinical examination and percutaneous biopsy is required to ensure that the screening process is specific. Following assessment, 3 out of 4 screening-provoked surgical procedures are for malignant disease. The sensitivity of screening mammography can be estimated by comparing the numbers of cancers occurring after a normal screening examination with the breast cancer incidence in a non-screened population. Such calculations show a 76% decrease in symptomatic breast cancer in the first year following a negative screen. This reduces to 41% and 21% in the second and third years after a negative screen (Day et al 1995).

Ultrasound

Breast ultrasound has the attractions of being both painless and ionizing radiation-free.

However, although sensitive in the detection of invasive malignancy it lacks sensitivity in the detection of DCIS (Ciatto et al 1994). Ultrasound of both breasts is time-consuming and the use of ultrasound to screen asymptomatic women currently has unacceptably low specificity. No randomized-controlled trial has shown a population mortality benefit from breast screening by ultrasound.

The evidence for the effectiveness of screening

Randomized controlled trials are the only reliable way of assessing any mortality benefit from screening. The first randomized-controlled trial of mammographic screening was the Health Insurance Plan (HIP) study (Shapiro et al 1988). More recent trials include the Swedish Two Counties, Edinburgh, Malmo, Stockholm and Gothenburg trials (Shapiro et al 1988, Nystrom et al 1993, Wald et al 1993, Bjurstam et al 1997). Four of these trials have shown statistically significant mortality reductions in all or at least some of the age groups screened. Meta-analysis of the combined results suggests a 22% reduction in mortality was achieved in the 40–74-year age range (relative risk 0.78, 95% CI 0.70–0.87) in those invited for screening. In women aged 50–74 the mortality reduction achieved in these trials was 24% (RR 0.76, 95% CI 0.67–0.87) (Wald et al 1993). The mortality reduction seen in women who actually attend for screening may be as high as 63% (Vitak et al 2001).

Number of views

All mammographic screens should include a cranio-caudal and medio-lateral oblique view of each breast. The one-view two-view trial showed that two-view mammography detects 24% more cancers with a 15% lower recall rate (Wald et al 1995). The costs per cancer found were similar whether one or two views were used. Two-view mammography leads to a 54% increase in detection of invasive cancer <10 mm in size. Such tumours are those most likely to lead to the mortality benefit associated with screening.

Number of readers

Double reading has the advantage of detecting more cancers but at the possible cost of increasing recall rates. Recent data from the NHSBSP indicate that double reading with arbitration is superior to independent double reading or double reading with consensus. Double reading with arbitration leads to a 32–40% increase in detection of small invasive cancers without increasing the recall rate (Blanks et al 1998). With the introduction of full-field digital mammography, computer-aided diagnosis (CAD) becomes a realistic option. CAD is particularly good at detecting microcalcifications (Jiang et al 1996). It remains to be seen if single reading with CAD is as effective as double reading.

Frequency of screening

The screening interval (the time between screening examinations) should be less than the lead-time provided by screening. (Lead-time is the time between diagnosis by screening and the time the cancer would have presented clinically.) If the screening interval is too long many interval cancers occur leading to a reduction in the effectiveness of screening. Estimates of the lead-time achieved by mammographic screening in women aged 40–49, 50–59 and 60–69 are 1.7, 3.3 and 3.8 years respectively (Tabar et al 1995). A sharp increase in interval cancers is observed in the third year after screening compared with the first and second years after screening (Burrell et al 1996). Particularly high interval cancer rates are seen in younger women. These facts suggest that a 12-month screening interval in women under 50 and a 2-year interval in women over 50 are likely to be the most effective.

Age

The combined Swedish results show a significant mortality reduction in women aged 50–59 and 60–69 (RR reduction of 28% and 31% respectively) (Nystrom et al 1993). Two factors also indicate that screening is cost-effective in this age group. Firstly, there is a high breast cancer incidence in this age group (at least two times that in women aged 40–49) and, secondly, the lead time of screening in this age group is such that the screening interval does not need to be less than 2 years.

The initial results of the randomized trials did not show a significant mortality reduction in women aged 40–49. However, recent results from the Malmo and Gothenburg trials show statistically significant mortality reductions in women under 50 of 36% and 45% respectively (Bjurstam et al 1997). Both these trials used modern mammography, a short screening interval and at least five screening rounds.

Lower prevalence-to-incidence ratios and a shorter time to natural incidence of breast cancer after a negative screen in women under 50 indicate a shorter lead-time. This suggests that the interval between screens should be shorter in younger women. Annual or 18-monthly mammography is required when screening women under 50. Although screening women under 50 has now been shown to be effective, the low incidence of breast cancer in women under 50 and the frequency of screening required means that screening women under 50 may not be cost-effective.

The combined Swedish results did not show a mortality benefit from screening in women aged 70–74. This result was probably due to poor attendance. There is therefore no clear evidence to support screening women aged over 70 years.

Recall for assessment

Multidisciplinary assessment of screen-detected abnormalities is required to confirm benignity or malignancy quickly and efficiently. Recall for assessment causes considerable anxiety so it is important that the recall rate is kept as low as possible without compromising sensitivity. Recall rates in the NHSBSP should be less than 7% in the prevalent round and less than 5% at incident screens. The anxiety caused by recall is usually short-term and rarely has long-standing consequences. Abnormalities requiring recall should have a >5% chance of being malignant, these include ill-defined masses, speculate mass,

distortion and suspicious calcifications. Most asymmetric densities and well-defined masses do not require recall.

Assessment

Assessment should be carried out by a multidisciplinary team including a radiologist, clinician, pathologist, radiographer and breast care nurse. Patients normally undergo further imaging initially. Clinical examination is then performed in those women where further imaging has confirmed the presence of a significant abnormality.

Core biopsy is carried out in those women where a significant abnormality is confirmed. Percutaneous needle biopsy is usually carried out under imaging guidance and is best carried out using ultrasound guidance. Stereotaxis is required for lesions such as calcification, which are often not visible on ultrasound. Digital stereotaxis is particularly useful when biopsying microcalcification (Whitlock et al 2000). Specimen x-rays are used to confirm adequate sampling of microcalcifications. Five flecks of calcium or three cores containing calcification on the specimen x-ray enable accurate non-operative diagnosis (Bagnall et al 2000). Digitally acquired specimen x-rays enable the number of cores taken to be tailored to the individual.

Vacuum-assisted mammotomy is a method for obtaining larger volumes of tissue compared to core. Its main indication is to biopsy microcalcification especially cases that are technically difficult to sample with core biopsy. The main disadvantage of vacuum-assisted mammotomy is cost, the disposables being 10–15 times the cost of automated core biopsy or needles. There is the risk with this technique removing the whole radiological abnormality. Deployment of a metallic clip to aid future localization is often required (Philpotts et al 1999).

The estimate of risk of malignancy of a lesion is based on the combination of imaging and clinical findings. Patient management is based on the most suspicious of these findings. Lesions with a low risk of malignancy are returned to normal screening on the basis of a definitively benign biopsy result. Lesions with a high risk of malignancy are sampled prior to surgical excision with the aim of making a pre-operative diagnosis of malignancy so therapeutic surgery can be facilitated. Preoperative diagnosis rates for malignancy of >90% for invasive disease and 75% for DCIS disease can be achieved using core biopsy.

Patient management is best decided at a prospective multidisciplinary meeting where the pathological, imaging and clinical findings are discussed prior to the woman's follow-up appointment. Women should either be returned to normal screening or have surgical removal of the lesion. Short-term recall is associated with psychological morbidity, making it a less-favoured option.

Localization biopsies

Over 50% of screen-detected abnormalities requiring removal for therapeutic or diagnostic purposes will be impalpable and will require marker localization. Marker localizations are usually performed using a wire. Skin marking, carbon granules and isotopes may also be used. Marker localization is best performed under ultrasound guidance but stereotaxis is required for lesions not visible on ultrasound.

Quality assurance

For breast cancer screening to be effective a high standard of performance must be achieved by all facets of the service. From its inception the NHSBSP has had quality assurance guidelines for all aspects of the service including radiography, equipment, radiology, pathology and surgery. Quality assurance guidelines for radiologists include cancer detection rates, small cancer detection rates, recall rates, benign biopsy rates and preoperative diagnosis rates (NHSBSP 1997). All units submit information regularly to regional quality assurance centres. Multidisciplinary quality assurance visits occur regularly and audit all aspects of a unit's performance. Areas of poor performance are identified and must be shown to have been corrected at follow-up visits.

REFERENCES

Bagnall MC, Evans AJ, Wilson ARM, Burrell H, Pinder SE. When have mammographic calcifications been adequately sampled at needle core biopsy. *Clinical Radiology* 2000; **55**: 548–553.

Bjurstam N, Bjorneld L, Duffy SW, et al. The Gothenburg Breast Screening Trial. First results on mortality, Incidence and mode of detection for women ages 39–49 years at randomization. *Cancer* 1997; **80**: 2091–2099.

Blanks RG, Wallis MG, Moss SM. A comparison of cancer detection rates achieved by breast cancer screening programmes by number of readers, for one and two view mammography: results from the National Health Service breast screening programme. *Journal of Medical Screening* 1998; **5**: 195–201.

Burrell HC, Sibbering DM, Wilson ARM, et al. The mammographic features of interval cancers and prognosis compared with screen detected and symptomatic breast cancers. *Radiology* 1996; **199**: 811–817.

Ciatto S, Rosselli Del Turco M, Catarzi S, Morrone D. The contribution of ultrasonography to the differential diagnosis of breast cancer. *Neoplasma* 1994; **41**: 341–345.

Day N, McCann J, Camilleri-Ferrante C, et al. Monitoring interval cancers in breast screening programmes: the East Anglian experience. *Journal of Medical Screening* 1995; **2**: 180–185.

Ellman R, Moss S, Coleman D, Chamberlain J. Breast self examination programmes in the early detection of breast cancer. *British Journal of Cancer* 1993; **68**: 208–212.

Jiang Y, Nishikawa RM, Wolverton DE, et al. Malignant and benign clustered microcalcifications: Automated feature analysis and classification. *Radiology* 1996; **198**: 671–678.

NHSBSP. Quality assurance guidelines for radiologists. May 1997.

Nystrom L, Rutqvist L, Wall S, et al. Breast cancer screening with mammography; overview of Swedish randomised trials. *Lancet* 1993; **341**: 973–978.

Philpotts LE, Shaheen NNA, Lange RC, Lee CH. Comparison of rebiopsy rates after stereotactic core needle biopsy of the breast with 11-gauge vacuum suction probe versus 14-gauge needle and automatic gun. *American Journal of Roentgenology* 1999; **172**: 683–687.

Shapiro S, Venet W, Strax P, Venet L. Periodic screening for breast cancer: the Health Insurance Plan project and its sequelae, 1963–1986. London: Johns Hopkins University Press, 1988.

Tabar L, Fagerberg G, Chen H, Duffy S, Gad A. Screening for breast cancer in women aged under 50: mode of detection, incidence, fatality, and histology. *Journal of Medical Screening* 1995; **2**: 94–98.

Tabar L, Vitak B, Chen HT, et al. Beyond Randomised Controlled Trials. *Cancer* 2001; **91**: 1724–1731.

Wald NJCJ, Hackshaw A. Consensus Statement. Report of the European Society for Mastology Breast Cancer Screening Evaluation Committee (1993). *The Breast* 1993; **2**: 209–216.

Wald N, Murphy P, Major P, Parkes C, Townsend J, Frost C. UKCCCR multicentre randomised controlled trial of one and two view mammography in breast cancer screening. *British Medical Journal* 1995; **311**: 1189–1193.

Whitlock JPL, Evans AJ, Burrell HC, Pinder SE, Ellis IO, Blamey RW, Wilson ARM. Digitally acquired imaging improves upright stereotactic core biopsy of mammographic microcalcifications. *Clinical Radiology* 2000; **55**: 374–377.

13

Psychological issues and communication

This chapter provides an outline of:

- breast cancer and anxiety,
- communication skills and anxiety reduction,
- role of the mammography practitioner,
- breast cancer and the family.

BREAST CANCER AND ANXIETY

Women attend a mammography service for a variety of reasons. They may be referred by their doctor with a potentially significant breast symptom or they may be part of a screening programme. The screening programme could be national, local, part of a research project, a pilot project or for family history. Women may be attending for further investigation of an abnormality identified at screening or they may have had a diagnosis and treatment for breast cancer and be on post treatment surveillance. Whatever the reason, those attending the service are likely to have some anxieties in common. They may be concerned about radiation dose or that the procedure may be painful and/or embarrassing. More significantly they will be affected by fear of the potential outcome.

Breast cancer is a highly emotive disease. The word cancer still brings with it a sense of potential mortality. Despite advances in disease treatment and earlier diagnosis, cancer remains a major threat to life. Mortality resulting from circulatory diseases has decreased significantly in the last 5 years, but mortality from cancer has not decreased at a similar rate. In the case of breast cancer, despite early diagnosis and improved treatments, mortality rates, although reducing, still remain comparatively high. Apart from raising anxiety relating to personal mortality and the impact this may have on family and friends, a diagnosis of breast cancer also brings with it the potential for disfiguring surgery.

Many women who attend for diagnostic procedures will have a benign outcome, however, all will experience similar fears and anxieties until the final outcome is known. Fear and anxiety are natural processes which prepare us for fight or flight. When confronted with a potential threat this primeval drive comes into play. The anxieties relating to a possible breast cancer diagnosis, once triggered, will remain with the individual for some time after the all clear, and in screening this is viewed as a negative effect of the screening process. For the health care professional dealing with the woman there will be some sense of the likely significance of a clinical sign or mammographic abnormality. However, for the patient these factors have no significance and each is fearful for themselves and their families. It is important that all health care professionals are aware of this and are alert and sensitive to individual needs.

The anxiety experienced, and how it is manifested, will vary from individual to individual. Each individual will also have differing coping styles. Some women will want their partners with them throughout; others may well prefer to deal with the process alone until the outcome is known. Whatever the coping style, there will be anxiety but it may be well hidden. All staff need to be sensitive to this and recognize that this may influence behaviour patterns.

Women who have previously been given a cancer diagnosis and had treatment for the disease will generally be placed on regular follow-up for several years after diagnosis. Their fears will differ to some degree from those in the pre-diagnostic phase. They will already have faced a cancer diagnosis and considered their own mortality. They will have drawn on their defences and dealt with the immediate issues. However, these women have to live with cancer for the rest of their life and this may have long-term effects on their psychological well being and

their quality of life. The majority of women who have previously been diagnosed and treated for breast cancer will have been offered the support of a counselling nurse and/or therapy counsellor at diagnosis and through the treatment phase. Women may decline this psychological support in the early stages but may require it at a later stage. Health care professionals involved in patient follow up should be alert to signs that psychological support may be needed and report their concerns to the appropriate members of the team.

REDUCING ANXIETY

A woman receiving an invitation to screening or considering visiting a general practitioner to seek referral for a breast symptom will already have been subject to a plethora of information relating to breast cancer. She may have had first-hand experience when a family member or close friend has suffered from breast cancer or she may have friends who have had first-hand experience. She will also have inevitably been subject to vast amounts of information in women's newspapers, magazines, television, radio, films and the internet. Some of this information will be accurate and some inaccurate. These experiences and accumulated knowledge will inevitably colour the patient's perception of the disease and its likely outcome. It may also affect her attitude on attendance at the breast clinic. Anxiety levels will also be influenced by her own personality together with the phase of her relationship with the disease of breast cancer.

Multiple phases of the disease have been identified. It can be assumed that there is a direct relationship between anxiety and the quality of life, in that the worse the quality of life then the greater the degree of anxiety, and vice versa. Given this assumption, then an approximate indication of the various anxiety levels associated with different phases of the disease can be appreciated (**Table 13.1**). About a third of women who have a newly diagnosed cancer suffer from anxiety and depression, and this incidence almost doubles over the next 3 months as the realization of the seriousness of the diagnosis and its implications become apparent. Particularly at risk are those

Table 13.1 The phases of a woman's relationship with breast cancer, showing the de Haes quality of life scores (0–100) and an estimate of anxiety levels

Phase of relationship with breast cancer	Quality of life score (de Haes)	Estimate of anxiety level
Complete ignorance	–	0
Relative or friend with breast cancer	–	5
Invitation to be screened	94	10
Breast symptom – especially a lump	–	12
Assessment of abnormality	–	13
Surgical biopsy	71	14
Treatment by local excision	74	13
Treatment by mastectomy	64	15
Disease-free interval (local excision)	83	12
Disease-free interval (mastectomy)	80	12
Living with metastases (depends on therapy)	30–60	16–33
Terminal phase	17	58

The estimate of anxiety level is calculated as 1000 times the reciprocal of the de Haes median score (de Haes et al 1993).

women who have an asymptomatic cancer identified, and to whom the diagnosis is made known over a short time scale. The speed of transference from 'I am normal' to 'I have a life-threatening disease' is critical. For a woman to have some prior indication of the possible diagnosis before it is actually confirmed seems to be associated with less long-term psychiatric morbidity. Almost two-thirds of women who have had a biopsy, with either a benign or malignant diagnosis, suffer from anxiety and depression. After 3 months about half of them are still affected. Following the treatment of breast cancer a steady incidence occurs in one fifth of women (**Table 13.2**).

Written information

One way of helping reduce anxiety is to provide written information for women who are attending prior to their arrival. Breast screening

Table 13.2 Incidence of anxiety and depression in groups of women in different phases of relationship with breast cancer

	Initial (%)	After 3 months (%)
Routine screening	25	19
False positive	30	19
Newly diagnosed cancer	34	46
Biopsied	59	37.5
Post-treatment	21	21
Symptomatic benign disease	35	31

After Ellman et al 1989.

programmes should take considerable care to provide suitable and accurate information for women invited to attend. This generally provides sufficient information about the risks and benefits of screening and something about the test itself. This places the invitation into a factually accurate context and enables women to make an informed decision. Other breast diagnostic services should also provide some written information relating to the appropriate clinic whether this be symptomatic, family history or follow up. Information included might be waiting times, what to wear, where to park, who can come with them, likely tests and the professional team. All of these can help reduce anxiety about the process and procedures and may go some way towards putting their individual risk into some degree of rational and understandable perspective. Letters can be supplemented by leaflets providing some additional information and perhaps repeating key messages placed in the letter.

Waiting times

Waiting is a great exacerbate of anxiety. Appointment times must be honoured and all the waiting periods between different stages of a consultation should be kept to an absolute minimum. A woman should be informed of the reason for, and the likely duration of any delays. In the case of one-stop clinics where a series of diagnostic tests may be performed, women should be advised of the process together with the potential delays and benefits.

Administrative and reception staff

The importance of skilful reception staff should not be underestimated. Women may contact the unit by telephone for a variety of enquiries. In many services they will also be the first representatives of the team to meet the woman on attendance. It is helpful if reception staff have some knowledge and understanding of the anxieties women may experience and how to deal with them. It is also important that reception staff feel able to alert other staff to potential problems and to call on other staff to deal with specific issues. This will enable reception staff to respond to patient needs in a truly effective way and to enable them to recognize patients who may need additional support.

The multiprofessional clinical team

The diagnosis and management of breast cancer is based on a multidisciplinary approach. The team includes radiographers, radiologists, surgeons, nurses and clinical support staff. All professions involved in delivering the service have a role to play in supporting women through the process. The value of good communication skills should never be underestimated. Every individual who comes into contact with the women can contribute to improving their psychological well being. A woman must gain the firm impression that the whole team is competent clinically and supportive emotionally.

Communication is of paramount importance. A woman should be given a full explanation of what any procedure entails before it is performed and it should be ensured that she understands. At the conclusion she should be told when the results will be available, and how they will be communicated to her. Information regarding the results should be simply and frankly explained, preferably by a doctor, who should also make her aware of the implications. Again it should be ensured that she understands this explanation.

Women who are finally given a diagnosis of cancer should always be provided with expert emotional support. Common practice is for 'bad news' to be given by a doctor with a breast care or counselling nurse in attendance. The discussion with the doctor is still regarded as the most significant communication for the patient, but the expert counsellor can help clarify several issues and will be trained to identify psychological cues which may indicate that the patient is not coping well.

MAMMOGRAPHY PRACTITIONERS AND COMMUNICATION

Different types of mammography examinations are likely to raise anxiety levels by differing degrees. The least worrying mammogram for a woman will be one taken as part of routine screening, but even so 25% of screened women will have measurable levels of anxiety and depression associated with the examination. This incidence falls to normal by 3 months after the screening episode. Women who are recalled for assessment, but are then found to be normal,

Table 13.3 Mammographic procedures likely to have an exacerbating effect on existing anxiety levels

	Increasing effect
Screening mammogram	
Family history surveillance	
Post-treatment follow-up examination (after the first)	
Diagnostic mammogram	↓
Image-guided core-cut or fine needle aspiration	
Diagnostic marker biopsy	
First post-treatment follow up examination	
Post-treatment examination with further symptoms	

have a slightly higher (30%) incidence of measurable anxiety, but this too falls to normal levels by 3 months. A routine screening mammogram is likely to have a lower exacerbating effect than special views taken for the elucidation of a problem, and much lower than mammography-guided fine needle aspiration or core cut sampling (**Table 13.3**).

All those individuals who are involved in breast disease diagnosis and management will inevitably have their attitudes influenced by breast cancer. Resulting from the increased importance of mammography in the management of breast cancer, mammographers are now pre-eminent in this group. Therein lies a benefit and a danger. Being aware of the background, a mammographer can more readily appreciate the woman's attitude to her problems. However, the mammographer should realize that his/her own perceptions are affected and should not identify too closely with the woman. He/she should maintain a professional attitude and a degree of authority.

The mammographer is placed in very close physical contact with a woman during the examination; not only is there potential embarrassment and a significant 'intrusion into personal space' but the technique required to perform a mammogram can be likened to an embrace. It follows that this degree of intimacy places a particular responsibility upon the mammographers who should be sensitive to the psychological state of the woman, and be prepared to give whatever support may be necessary. To accomplish this it is essential to perform the examination in an efficient, confident manner, being as physically gentle as is consistent with the production of a high-quality mammogram, and simultaneously expressing obvious empathy and a caring attitude.

It is also due to the intimacy of the examination that women may bring issues previously hidden, to the fore. These may be issues of a personal nature and in a routine screening examination this can be quite a common occurrence. It provides a chance for the woman to talk to someone fully and frankly about an issue which they will not necessarily share with others. In examinations where anxiety levels relate to breast cancer (**Table 13.1**) the woman may openly express these fears.

Personal issues

Radiographers and other mammography practitioners are trained to be experts in the area of clinical practice. This puts the mammographer at an advantage over the women. She is likely to perceive the practitioner as more powerful and in order to undertake the test will generally be compliant with the requests of the mammographer and have respect for their professional expertise. When an issue of a personal nature is brought to the mammographer's attention it is important to remember that in this area the mammographer is no longer the expert. There is essentially a change in dynamics of the relationship. As a practitioner performing an examination the mammographer is the expert, in terms of personal lives only the patient can be the expert.

Although as a general rule mammographers do not act as professional counsellors, on occasions they are called upon to use counselling skills. It is important to remember that counselling skills rely heavily on listening skills and the use of open questions. For the woman, the expression of and verbalization of the issue may well be what provides the relief, albeit temporarily, to the problem raised. The strength of the relationship with the mammographer is that she/he is independent of their normal life, will respect confidentiality and will not judge. The mammographer in this situation should not give advice but simply listen, reflect and clarify.

Breast cancer issues

Given the intimacy of mammography and that it is often the first clinical test performed, anxieties about the outcome may be expressed very readily. Information that the woman has not requested should not be offered. However, eliciting whether more information is required is entirely appropriate and leaves the choice to the women. This allows the woman to seek information but only when she is ready to cope with potential answers. To ask 'Is there anything you need to know about . . .' will often precipitate a question which the woman has not completely formulated previously, or is reticent to ask. In a breast screening follow-up situation, a frequently asked question is why they have been recalled. This can often be answered by showing the original screening films. This should be left to experienced mammographers who can show the films without being drawn on the potential outcome. The women can then see the difference from one side to the other, realize the importance of having this area checked out and understand why no answers are immediately available. This knowledge will also help to explain why certain procedures are required and that any associated discomfort is necessary.

It is important that the mammographer is aware of the limitations of his/her role and is not drawn to answer questions for which there is, as yet, no answer. Telling the woman when and how she will get the answers to these questions can be extremely helpful. It cannot be overstressed that great care is necessary before suggesting to a woman that the diagnosis is, or may be, cancer. Communication with the woman on this topic is best left to those who are able to provide the full clinical facts, can discuss the choices available and have the necessary counselling training to fully support the woman. This can put enormous pressure on the mammographer. In the meantime, a balance is needed in which neither too much nor too little reassurance is offered.

The mammographer can help women through the various stages of the diagnosis, and treatment when treatment is necessary, by being alert to the individual needs of the women and addressing these to the best of their ability within the context of a multiprofessional team.

THE FAMILY

It has been established for many years that a woman's ability to cope with her anxieties relates strongly to the degree of support she receives. Husbands, partners and close family members are identified as primary sources of support. Self-help groups, such as the Mastectomy Association and voluntary support groups serve as visible evidence that problems and fears can be overcome. Breast cancer is a family disease. The supportive role of a family has been referred to above, but the full effect of a diagnosis of breast cancer on the family may not always be fully appreciated. There is no doubt that healthy family members can be affected by the illness of another family member, with the creation of physical, emotional and social symptoms. Moreover, the way one family member reacts to an illness can affect the way that another member adjusts. With breast cancer in particular, family members may have considerable difficulty in coping with the emotional ramifications. The occurrence of problems is likely to be greatest during the first year after the development of metastases. Every individual working in a breast diagnostic service has a responsibility to be aware of the problems. The attitude and state of mind of the husband or other family member who accompanies a woman scheduled to have diagnostic tests merits careful consideration. A sympathetic and supportive attitude should be extended to accompanying persons as and when this is judged to be appropriate.

FURTHER READING

Aro AR, de Koning HJ, Absetz P, Schreck M. Psychological predictors of first attendance for organised mammography screening. *Journal of Medical Screening* 1999; **6**(2): 82–88.
Aro HR, Polvikki Absetz S, van Elderen TM, van der Ploeg E et al. False positive findings in mammography screening induces short-term distress – breast cancer specific concern prevails longer. *European Journal of Cancer* 2000; **36**(9): 1089–1097.
Austoker J. Gaining informed consent for screening. Is difficult-but many misconceptions need to be undone. *British Medical Journal* 1999; **319**(7212): 722.

Austoker J, Ong G. Written information needs of women who are recalled for further investigation of breast screening: results of a multi centre study. *Journal of Medical Screening* 1994; **1**(4): 238–244.

Bryla CM. The relationship between stress and the development of breast cancer: a literature review. *Oncology Nursing Forum* 1996; **23**(3): 441–448.

Cancer Trends in England and Wales 1950–1999. *www.statistics.gov.uk*

Cancer Survival 1992–1999. *www.statistics.gov.uk*

Dean C, Roberts MM, French K, Robinson S. Psychiatric morbidity after screening for breast cancer. *Journal of Epidemiology and Community Health* 1986; **42**: 1239–1241.

de Haes JCJM, de Koning HJ. Quality of life and breast cancer screening. In: Gad A, Rosselli del Turco M, eds. *Breast Cancer Screening in Europe*. Berlin: Springer Verlag, 1993; 143–148.

Ellman R, Angeli N, Christians A, Moss S, Chamberlain J, Maguire PP. Psychiatric morbidity associated with screening for breast cancer. *British Journal of Cancer* 1989; **60**: 781–784.

Hafslund B, Mammography and the experience of pain and anxiety. *Radiography* 2000; **6**: 269–272.

Indicators of the Nations Health: Female death rates by selected causes. *www.dog.gsi.gov.uk.HPSSS*

Jamison KR, Wellish DK, Passnau RO. Psychosocial aspects of mastectomy: 1. The woman's perspective. *American Journal of Psychiatry* 1978; **135**: 543–546.

Lowe J, Balanda KP, Del Mar C, Hawes E. Psychological distress in women with abnormal findings in mass mammography screening. *Cancer* 1999; **85**(5): 1114–1118.

MacVicar M. The effect of cancer in the male spouse on the family. *Dissertation Abstracts International* 1976; **36**: 5582A.

Maguire P, Parkes CM. Surgery and loss of body parts. *British Medical Journal* 1998; **316**: 1086–1088.

Minuchin S. *Families and Family Therapy*. Cambridge, Massachusetts: Harvard University Press, 1974.

Northouse LL. The impact of cancer in women on the family. *Cancer Practitioner* 1995; **3**(3): 134.

Ong G, Austoker J. Recalling women for further investigation of breast screening: women's expediencies at the clinic and afterwards. *Journal of Public Health and Medicine* 1997; **19**(1): 29–36.

Poole K, Lyne PA. The 'cues' to diagnosis: describing the monitoring activities of women undergoing diagnostic investigations for breast disease. *Journal of Advanced Nursing* 2000; **31**(4): 752–758.

Scaf-Clomp W, Sanderman R, van de Weil HB Otter R et al. Distressed or relived? Psychological side effects of breast cancer screening in the Netherlands. *Journal of Epidemiology and Community Health* 1997; **51**(6): 705–710.

Seckel MM, Birney MH. Social support, stress and age in women undergoing breast biopsies. *Clinical Nurse Specialist* 1996; **10**(3): 137–143.

Steggles S, Lightfoot N, Sellick SM Psychological distress associated with organised breast cancer screening. *Cancer Prevention and Control* 1998; **2**(5): 213–220.

Trief PM, Khan S. Assessing emotional distress of women with breast cancer: a survey of clinical oncologists. *Breast Cancer Res Treatment* 1997; **3**(3): 134–142.

Walker BL. Adjustment of husbands and wives to breast cancer. *Cancer Practitioner* 1997; **5**(2): 92–98.

Appendix 1

Quality control tests

It is important that all radiographers working in the unit take part in quality control tests and understand why they require to be carried out. There should be a designated person with responsibility for monitoring these checks and taking action when the results fall outwith tolerance levels. There must be clearly defined guidelines and written protocols to be followed when results indicate that no further examinations should be undertaken using that equipment. The decision to stop screening in an asymptomatic breast screening programme should lie with the clinical director in consultation with the quality assurance radiographer and the responsible medical physics department.

DAILY TESTS
Sensitometry

This is described in detail in **Chapter 2**. A sensitometric strip should be processed as soon as the processor reaches its normal working temperature to ensure that it is functioning correctly. The films of the 4 cm block should not be processed until this has been checked. A further sensitometry strip should be processed when the processor has been processing films for about an hour. It is the measurements on this film which should be entered on the control chart.

AEC consistency test

This is described in detail in **Chapter 1**. This should be carried out daily by the radiographer who is about to use that particular machine before any mammography is undertaken. The resultant density should be plotted on a graph. This density should not vary more than ± 0.15 OD from the present value. Should this occur, the first step to take is to repeat the sensitometry to ensure that the anomaly is not created by the processor. This should be followed by a repeat block test if the sensitometry is not out of tolerance. The decision to stop using the machine should be taken when the resulting density falls outwith the range 1.4–1.8 OD.

WEEKLY TESTS
AEC tests

The AEC should be tested using 2, 4 and 6/7 cm of perspex to ensure that it will produce the same densities irrespective of the tissue density in the beam.

Image quality phantom

A film should be taken of the image quality phantom each week and scored according to the instructions pertaining to the phantom which is used. This should be compared with the previous week and the 'GOLD STANDARD' which was taken on installation of the equipment. It is important that any deterioration is rectified before the mammographic image shows signs of degradation. It is easy to ignore small changes which occur slowly over time.

Stereotactic device

If the device is used frequently its accuracy should be checked weekly as described in the operator's manual. Should the device be used infrequently, then it should be checked before use.

Emergency switch off

The emergency switch off should be checked for function.

MONTHLY TESTS

Mechanical safety of the machine should be checked. All movements should be free running and there should be no over-running of any movement. All surfaces should be checked for rough edges.

QUARTERLY TESTS

- **Film screen contact,**
- **Absorption** and **output** from the screens.

PROCESSOR SERVICE

This should be carried out at 6-monthly intervals.

PATIENT SAFETY

It is the responsibility of all radiographers using any of the equipment to ensure that there are no sharp edges to injure the woman or the operator, that cables and cassettes are not wearing and that all emergency switches function correctly.

Appendix 2

Investigation protocols

This appendix provides a series of practical protocols:

- Section 1: Protocols for masses detected clinically,
- Section 2: protocols for lesions detected by mammography – masses, architectural distortions, calcifications. Each protocol relates to the estimate of risk.

GOLDEN RULES

- The object of investigating any breast abnormality is to determine the definitive diagnosis: with the least number of investigatory steps, with the minimum inconvenience to the patient, with the acquisition of a knowledge of all factors necessary for optimal management of the problem.
- There is absolutely no point whatsoever in undertaking investigations which will not alter the management of an individual patient, no matter how much better the additional investigation may demonstrate a particular lesion.
- Imaging investigations cannot make a definitive diagnosis, but can only indicate the probability of what the final diagnosis might be.
- Tissue diagnosis can be made preoperatively by fine needle aspiration (FNA) for cytology, or by core biopsy.
- The basis of investigation is the investigator's estimation of the final outcome, with the risk classified as:
  - benign,
  - probably benign,
  - indeterminate,
  - probably malignant,
  - malignant.
- When there are two disciplines involved, eg. clinician and radiologist, then the opinion with the highest risk takes precedence in determining the protocol to be adopted.

SECTION 1

ABNORMALITIES PRESENTING AS A PALPABLE MASS

STEP 1

When a palpable mass is to be investigated, the first step is for an experienced breast clinician to classify the lesion on a five-point risk scale:

1. benign,
2. probably benign,
3. indeterminate,
4. probably malignant,
5. malignant.

This will enable the investigations to be tailored to the particular problem confronting the woman.

PROTOCOL 'A'

Palpable masses classified by the clinician as benign

Management of this group depends on the age of the woman.

A woman under 35 years of age, when carcinoma is extremely uncommon, can be discharged with confidence if an **ultrasound examination and a freehand FNA or core biopsy** show no evidence of malignancy. Mammography is not indicated.

For women between the ages of 35 and 50, **ultrasound** is performed unless the lesion is thought to be solid, when a mammogram is undertaken.

For women over 50 years of age, when the incidence of cancer is becoming more significant, then **mammography** is the first investigation to be performed, followed by ultrasound.

Should imaging and the tissue diagnosis be classified as benign, then the woman may be discharged. If either the imaging or cytology/histology are classified as anything other than benign, then mammography is indicated (unless performed already).

Only if the combined imaging classification and tissue diagnosis are benign can the woman be discharged with confidence. Higher risk estimates necessitate moving to one of the next protocols.

Ultrasound

Following a study of all the characteristics of the lesion the ultrasonographer should classify the lesion on the five-point risk scale indicated above. Should this be benign no further imaging investigation is required, but in any other eventuality (probably benign through to malignant) then mammography is indicated.

Mammography

A full mammographic series (cranio-caudal and medio-lateral oblique projections of both sides) is required and a combined risk classification of the presenting lesion should be made on the basis of both the ultrasound and mammographic examinations.

FNA or core biopsy

FNA or core biopsy is best undertaken **freehand** or with **ultrasound** guidance.

PROTOCOL 'B'

Palpable masses classified by clinician as probably benign and indeterminate

Palpable mass lesions classified as probably benign or indeterminate will need to have a tissue diagnosis made by FNA or core biopsy. In addition, further investigation is indicated to characterize the lesion and to confirm the likelihood of malignancy in each individual case. **Ultrasound** is the first investigation of choice, since if the lesion is well demonstrated this is the most accurate method to obtain a tissue sample by FNA or core biopsy. **Mammograms** are required if both U/S and FNA do not indicate a benign condition. This will enable the radiologist to study both the lesion, the remainder of the breast and the contralateral breast.

Ultrasound

A study of all the characteristics of the lesion should be made, and the ultrasonographer should classify the lesion on the five-point risk scale indicated above. Should this be benign no further imaging investigation is required, but in any other eventuality (probably benign through to malignant) then mammography is indicated.

Mammography

A full mammographic series is required.

A combined risk classification of the presenting lesion should be made on the basis of both the U/S and mammographic examinations.

FNA or core biopsy

FNA or core biopsy is best undertaken **freehand** or with **ultrasound** guidance.

PROTOCOL 'C'

Palpable masses classified by clinician as probably malignant or malignant

Most lesions classified as probably malignant and all those as malignant are destined for open surgery. A preoperative tissue diagnosis will be made by fine needle aspiration (FNA) for cytology, or by core biopsy. Thus imaging investigations are directed towards obtaining information essential to the proper management of the case.

Mammogram

A pre-operative mammogram series (bilateral cranio-caudal and medio-lateral oblique projections) is performed, not only to assess the suspect lesion, but in the search for other lesions in the ipsi- or contra-lateral breast. The image of the suspect lesion is studied specifically for features which might have a bearing on treatment choice, such as an estimate of tumour size (mammography is more accurate in the estimation of tumour size than palpation) or the presence of associated DCIS.

Ultrasound

If freehand FNA is considered inadequate an ultrasound-guided FNA should be performed. Ultrasound should be performed as it can give a more accurate estimate of size than mammography and it should be considered if a precise pre-operative measurement is required. Ultrasound can also provide additional information about multifocality and tumour extent. Ultrasound is not required if the carcinoma is considered to be locally advanced. Ultrasound may also be helpful in imaging the axilla for significant lymphadenopathy

FNA or core biopsy

FNA or core biopsy can be undertaken **freehand** or with **ultrasound guidance**.

SECTION 2

MASS LESIONS DETECTED ON MAMMOGRAPHY

STEP 1

An experienced radiologist should classify the lesion on the five-point risk scale (benign, probably benign, indeterminate, probably malignant, and malignant). With the exception of those lesions classified as benign, these all require examination by a clinician. Should the clinical and radiological assessment of suspicion be at variance then the higher degree of suspicion determines the action.

PROTOCOL 'D'

Impalpable mass lesions classified by radiologist as benign

No further investigation is required for this group of conditions which includes such entities as masses with the characteristic 'popcorn' calcification of a fibroadenoma or solitary, well defined masses and multiple masses, all of which appear similar.

PROTOCOL 'E'

Impalpable mass lesions classified by radiologist as probably benign, indeterminate or probably malignant

These lesions will all require tissue diagnosis unless they prove to be cystic, but before any needling is undertaken the woman should have a **clinical examination** by an experienced clinician. In the case of the probably malignant cases, a surgeon would be appropriate, since there is a high probability that the woman will require surgical management. Should the lesion be impalpable, and if it is solid, then an image-guided **FNA or core biopsy** will be required.

It is appropriate to undertake an **U/S examination** before referral to the clinician, in order to identify cystic lesions. This will also ascertain whether an image-guided FNA or core biopsy is to be under U/S or stereotactic guidance should the lesion prove to be impalpable. Further **complementary mammographic** views or **supplementary techniques** can also be undertaken with benefit before referral. Preliminary investigation will preclude the possibility that the clinician will needle the lesion before the imaging investigations are completed. The clinician should be given a combined risk assessment based on all the examinations taken before referral.

Mammography

It is assumed that a full series of films (obliques and cranio-caudals of each breast) was taken at the time of the initial

examination. If this was not the case then these should be taken, together with a repeat of any substandard projections.

Coned compression views of the suspect lesion in two projections will often assist in diagnosis by demonstrating the margins of a lesion more clearly. Magnification is rarely of value in this circumstance.

Ultrasound

The main objective is to differentiate cystic from solid lesions, since all solid lesions will require FNA or core biopsy.

FNA or core biopsy

FNA or core biopsy is best undertaken with **ultrasound guidance**.

PROTOCOL 'F'

Impalpable mass lesions classified by the radiologist as malignant

Surgery, with a pre-operative tissue diagnosis if possible, is required for these lesions, no matter what the result of any other investigations. The essential preliminary **clinical examination** should ideally be undertaken by an experienced surgeon since all these lesions will have to have surgery. As in the case of lesions classified as probably benign, indeterminate and probably malignant, it may well be of benefit to undertake preliminary **complementary mammography using supplementary techniques**, together with an **U/S examination** before the woman is seen by the surgeon.

Mammography

It is assumed that a full series of films (cranio-caudal and medio-lateral oblique projections of each breast) was taken at the time of the initial examination. If this was not the case then further views should be taken, together with a repeat of any substandard projections. **Coned compression** views of the suspect lesion in two projections will often assist in diagnosis by demonstrating the margins of a mass lesion more clearly. Magnification is rarely of value in this circumstance, unless calcifications are present within or in close association with the mass.

Ultrasound

The main objective is to differentiate cystic from solid lesions, since all solid lesions will require FNA or core biopsy. Lesions not seen on ultrasound should be treated as solid.

FNA or core biopsy

FNA or core biopsy is best undertaken with **ultrasound guidance**, or with x-ray guidance if not visible on ultrasound.

LESIONS PRESENTING AS ARCHITECTURAL DEFORMITIES DETECTED ON MAMMOGRAPHY

This is a difficult group of conditions to diagnose pre-operatively with accuracy. The presence of several radiographic signs may increase the probability that a particular lesion is benign or malignant, but all experienced radiologists are aware of cases when a sign which occurs most frequently in benign lesions (such as a 'white star') has been identified in a lesion proven to be malignant. Conversely, signs suggestive of malignancy (such as a 'black star') have occurred in lesions proven to be benign. In any individual case, therefore, one cannot be certain of the nature of the lesion.

The characteristics of this group of lesions when viewed by microscopy are of relatively few malignant cells, mostly confined to the periphery, with fibrosis and distorted normal tissues forming the bulk of the lesion. FNA and even core biopsy are therefore quite likely to miss the malignant cells and obtain only benign tissues. In spite of this, pre-operative tissue diagnosis should be attempted since a positive for malignancy will obviate the necessity for two operations, one a biopsy to establish the diagnosis, followed by a second to treat the condition should it prove to be cancer. Moreover, if a diagnosis can be made preoperatively, it will enable the woman to be counselled with appropriate treatment choices being offered.

In contradistinction to the difficulty of making a pre-operative diagnosis, to make the management decision is easy. **All architectural distortions require excision**.

Mammography

The main objective is to confirm that the architectural distortion is genuine, and not due simply to superimposition of normal tissues. It is assumed that a full series of films (obliques and cranio-caudals of each breast) was taken at the time of the initial examination. If this was not the case then further views should be taken, together with a repeat of any substandard projections.

Coned compression views of the suspect lesion, in two projections, will often assist in diagnosis by demonstrating the details and extent of the lesion more clearly. **Magnification** is sometimes of value in the investigation of architectural distortions, and may reveal unsuspected calcifications or other abnormality in close association with the lesion.

For this reason the technique of choice is **coned compression views with magnification**.

Ultrasound

U/S is unlikely to add any additional information.

FNA or core biopsy

FNA or core biopsy should be undertaken with **x-ray guidance**, and should be performed in the projection which best demonstrates the lesion.

LESIONS PRESENTING AS CALCIFICATIONS DETECTED ON MAMMOGRAPHY

To classify calcifications on the five-point risk scale is one of the greatest challenges to a radiologist. To facilitate this task it is essential that the radiography is of the very highest calibre. The appearance of the individual particles, the relationship of the particles to each other, and, if the particles are clustered together, the shape of the clusters themselves, are all important in the separation of benign from malignant lesions. One other feature which is important is the actual number of calcific particles, and whether the number visible increases on magnification.

Tissue diagnosis will be required unless the lesion is classified as benign. In some cases a follow-up examination after an interval might be of value. In this event the interval should not be less than 6 months, and one of a year is usually to be preferred.

Mammography

It is virtually mandatory to use **magnification** in the elucidation of calcifications, and in order to improve sharpness a small cone should be used. Thus the technique of choice is **coned compression views with magnification**. A two-view technique should be employed and it is essential that one of the projections should be with **a horizontal x-ray beam**, in order to demonstrate the 'tea cup' sign.

Ultrasound

U/S is unlikely to add any additional information.

FNA or core biopsy

FNA or core biopsy should be undertaken with **x-ray guidance**, and directed to that portion of the lesion in which the calcifications appear to be most likely to be associated with malignancy. Vacuum-assisted mammotomy is particularly helpful for the diagnosis of indeterminate microcalcifications.

Glossary

ANDI: Aberrations of normal development and involution. Otherwise known as benign breast change (BBC). A group of conditions which arise as a result of minor variations in the normal processes of development activity and involution. They are entirely benign and are variants of normality.

Automatic exposure control (AEC): A device which limits a radiographic exposure to a predetermined level. This is achieved by means of an ionization chamber, the position of which can be varied by a radiographer.

Basement membrane: The fine membrane upon which the outermost layer of cells which form a duct or lobule are based. It has importance in determining if a cancer is invasive or not.

BBC: Benign breast change. Also known as aberrations of normal development and involution (ANDI). A group of conditions which arise as a result of minor variations in the normal processes of development activity and involution. They are entirely benign and are variants of normality.

Biopsy: The removal of a small sample of tissue so that the tissue diagnosis may be established by histological techniques.

Bucky: A film cassette holder which contains a moving grid.

Cytology: A method to achieve tissue diagnosis by microscopic study of the characteristics of the cells of which the tissue is comprised. The cells to be studied are usually obtained by aspiration from the lesion into a fine needle – fine needle aspiration (FNA).

Embrology: The study of the prenatal development of an organ or individual.

Epithelium: The collection of cells which line the ducts and lobules of the breast. The epithelial cells in breast lobules secrete milk during lactation.

EQA: External quality assurance. It is desirable that the quality of a system is assessed by techniques applied from without the system in addition to techniques operated internally.

Filter: A material inserted in the x-ray beam to alter the quality of the beam by removing x-rays of unwanted energy. In some machines more than one filter is available and may be selected manually or automatically. Filters in common use are made from molybdenum, aluminium, palladium and selenium.

Frozen section: A histological technique which involves rapid freezing of a biopsy specimen so that slices may be made for histological study. The technique allows slices to be made without the inevitable time lag which is entailed in the paraffin wax technique (see Histology). However, the accuracy of diagnosis is often significantly less than with the paraffin wax technique, and many centres no longer rely upon frozen sections.

Histology: A method to achieve tissue diagnosis by microscopic study of a fine section of the tissue. The fine section is sliced from a piece of tissue obtained from a core removed within a cutting needle (core biopsy), or from a piece of tissue removed surgically. The tissue specimen is embedded in paraffin wax to enable a fine slice to be obtained. To assist in the study, the slice of tissue is stained to demonstrate particular characteristics.

Hyperplasia: An increase in the size and/or number of cells within a tissue.

    Typical hyperplasia: when the increase is of cells which have identical characteristics to the original cells.

    Atypical hyperplasia: when the additional cells show some variation from the original type.

Image-guided procedure: A procedure conducted using either x-ray or ultrasound images, particularly to ensure accuracy in needle placement.

Invasive carcinoma: A carcinoma which is not confined by the basement membrane of the ducts or lobules.

In situ cancer: A cancer which has not breached the basement membrane of the ducts or lobules. Ductal *in situ* carcinoma (DCIS) originates in the ducts. Lobular carcinoma *in situ* (LCIS) originates in the lobules. There is some debate whether this latter should be regarded as a cancer or as a risk factor.

Metastasis: The spread of cancer to a site distant from the original focus. The spread of cancer to remote sites is normally via the blood stream. The most common sites for metastases in breast cancer are the bones, the liver and the lungs.

Multifocal: The simultaneous occurrence of cancer at several sites within the same breast.

Parenchyma: A term which includes both the glandular tissue of the breast and the supporting stroma. It is the nature of the parenchyma which determines the density of the breast as visualized on a mammogram.

Projection: A radiographic 'view', classified according to the direction of the x-ray beam. Thus in a mediolateral projection the beam passes from the medial to the lateral aspect.

    Complementary projection: An additional projection taken in addition to the standard projections. Usually required to improve demonstration of an abnormality detected on a standard projection or to overcome an unusual physical feature which precludes full demonstration of breast tissue. Often taken on the same occasion as the standard projections.

    Standard projection: A projection taken as the basis for all mammographic examination. There are two projections generally accepted as standard, the mediolateral oblique and the craniocaudal. Some centres include a lateral projection as standard.

Proliferation: An increase in the number of cells which form a part of an organ.

QA: Quality assurance. The application of techniques to ensure that a system (or individual) is performing to an optimal level.

QC: Qualtity control. The application of techniques to ensure that a piece of apparatus is performing at an optimal level.

Risk factor: A factor which is associated with an increased risk of the development of cancer. The factor does not necessarily have a causative role.

Sclerosis: The formation of fibrous tissue, as in a scar or as a reacion to a pathological process – sclerosing adenosis, for example.

Stereotactic device: A device to facilitate the positioning of a needle within a lesion. Stereotactic computations are used to position a needle guide through which a needle may be inserted into the breast either for aspiration of cells (FNA), or for the insertion of a marker for surgical biopsy.

Stereotaxis: A method to determine the position of a lesion or suspected lesion within the breast, by obtaining two projections at an angle (usually 30 degrees). The depth is computed by reference to the known angle between the projections and the measured horizontal distances.

Stroma: An inert tissue supporting glandular tissue. It is comprised of strands of fibrous tissue with fat cells interspersed between them. A specialized form of stroma which does participate in some pathophysiological processes forms a cuff which surrounds the breast ducts and the glandular lobules.

Supplementary technique: An additional technique undertaken to elucidate an abnormality demonstrated on a standard or complementary examination, in order to obtain additional diagnostic information. Magnification mamography is an example.

Terminal ducto-lobular unit (TDL): The active part of the breast glandular tissue, situated at the periphery of the branching ductal system. The site of origin of many benign and malignant processes.

Triple assessment: The process of investigation of a breast problem using radiological, clinical and pathology techniques in combination.

Index